The Jamaican Public Health System
from the 17th–21st Centuries

The Jamaican Public Health System from the 17th–21st Centuries

A POLICY AND STRUCTURAL PERSPECTIVE

ADELLA CAMPBELL

UNIVERSITY OF TECHNOLOGY, JAMAICA PRESS

First published in Jamaica
University of Technology, Jamaica Press
237 Old Hope Road
Kingston 6
E-mail: utechjapress@utech.edu.jm

© 2018 by Adella Campbell

All rights reserved. Published 2018

A catalogue record of this book is available from the
National Library of Jamaica.

ISBN: 978-976-96211-0-7 (print)

While every effort has been made, it has not always been possible to identify the sources of all photographs used, or to trace all copyright holders. Please do get in touch with any enquiries or any information relating to the photographs or the rights holder.

Cover and book design by Robert Harris
Set in Minion Pro 11/14.5 x 27

Printed in the United States of America

Contents

Foreword

I felt a great sense of pride when Dr Campbell invited me to write the foreword to this book. She began her journey on this very important piece of work as she pursued doctoral studies at Victoria University of Wellington New Zealand and I was then the Government Chief Nursing Officer of Jamaica. Our paths intersected as she sought to glean credible information for the scholarly work which has resulted in the production of this book.

The health care system in Jamaica has always been one in which scholars, policy makers, health planners, health economists, health care professionals and practitioners, and health care users all have a vested interest. This book comes at an opportune time as Dr Campbell has sought to cull the literature on the Jamaican health sector in such a way as to provide the reader with "insight" into the delivery of health care services to the Jamaican citizenry over the period from the seventeenth to the twenty-first centuries.

Although there are many pieces of information available, this book has the benefit of guiding the reader through a timeline of four centuries and situates the Jamaican health care system within the broader context of the country's development. She lays out concisely the geographical, demographical, political, social and health, economic, and environmental characteristics of the country. Dr Campbell then allows us to focus on the indigenous people of this country, the Spaniards and early British plantation system. She outlines some of the health challenges related to these eras and solutions used to address them.

Readers are then guided to a place where Dr Campbell illuminates our understanding of and appreciation for the event related to the development and the reform of the health system from the seventeenth to the twenty-first centuries. It not only makes for interesting reading but it helps to strengthen our understanding of the systems and processes that were at play in the earlier centuries. Furthermore it serves to elucidate the processes that have allowed for the evolution of health system to where it is today.

This book guides the reader through a most interesting aspect of health policy; that of health reform. Dr Campbell guides us through the modern health reform of the health sector by way of discussing in her usual style the establishment of the Health Regions, their structure and function. She speaks to reform in the health sector in 2007 and 2008 with the focus on the abolition of user fees in the public health sector.

Dr Campbell takes us through a very critical aspect of health service delivery, that of financing health care from the seventeenth to the twenty-first centuries. This section also elaborates on the colonial period, the charges for health service and reform in user fees. She addresses other funding initiatives which include the National Health Fund, The CHASE Fund, the divestment of health services, budgetary allocation and health insurance.

Lastly this book details the health service delivery system and utilisation of the health care system. Readers have an opportunity to understand the network of service delivery facilities available. This section further captures the salient issues related to the various types of health facilities (secondary, primary and tertiary) and further delineates the structure of the typical Primary Health Care System. Dr Campbell has taken care in focusing on a critical aspect of care delivery as she delineates the nursing structure in the public health system and also the patients' journey in accessing care through the health care system. Not to be ignored is the significant role that folk culture plays in the health seeking behaviours of our people. This too is captured in this book for the reader's consideration.

This book is a valuable asset to all who have a keen interest in the health sector either from the position of a user, a provider, a policy maker or as an implementer of health policy. *The Jamaican Health Care System from the 17th–21st Centuries: A Policy and Structural Perspective* is written by one of our colleagues who, for the past seven years has been immersed in understanding the related policies and structures that have impacted the health care system in Jamaica. Her thorough and painstaking approach in consulting the work of others has allowed her to produce this seminal piece of work to make a lasting contribution to the history of available information on the health care system in Jamaica. This book will prove worthwhile to all those who have vested or even passing interest in the public health sector and its organisational and delivery system.

Leila McWhinney-Dehaney, PhD, MPH, FNP, RN RM,
Chairman, The Nursing Council of Jamaica

Preface

As a Commonwealth Scholar in New Zealand, I had to study the Jamaican Public Health System in depth in order to extrapolate from it various arrangements and collide these arrangements with the user fees policy which was the focus of my work at the time. If you have studied overseas, then you will identify with what I am about to share regarding my motivation for publishing this work. Of course, this is where I became acutely aware that there was a dearth of published work on the topic of interest. Further, there was no single text, writing or online resource which chronicled the development of the Jamaican Public Health System. This highlighted the need for a text of this nature.

As part of my work, therefore, I embarked on this venture of attempting to capture the Jamaican Public Health System in a booklet. This text elucidates the policies and structures which form the core of health infrastructure from one century to another. While this text may not provide all the details, it provides sufficient information that is in overwhelming demand by health practitioners, students in the health field, scholars, policymakers and the enquiring public. Generally, information contained in this text may be utilised in education, practice, research, policy development or for ones reading pleasure. Of note, this work is an extract from my 2013 dissertation and situation may have changed in some areas in the public health system.

The text provides a brief description of Jamaica as a country, then chronicles the development of the Jamaican Public Health System from the 17th century to the 21st century. It provides a framework for examining the sector from the Plantation System to reform of the health system in the 21st century. It provides context on the financing of the sector, health service delivery and utilisation, as well as the patients' journey as they traverse the system in a bid to access care. The Jamaican culture is very diverse and as such the influence of folklore has been included. This has been particularly important especially due to the fact that a number of individuals, despite utilising the conventional health system was also engaged in alternative therapy. The importance of the inextricable link between our history and our achievements to date in the health sector, is clearly highlighted in a reader-friendly manner.

Utilising an eclectic approach, information was extracted from several sources and weaved into this coherent whole and as such, I am indebted to the authors whose work I used. It was indeed a challenge but the importance of this work can be appreciated because of the relevance, appropriateness and usefulness of the information contained therein.

Acknowledgements

I must acknowledge divine guidance, without which this journey would have been futile. Profound thanks to my supervisors Dr Katherine Nelson and Associate Professor Jackie Cumming for the tremendous support and guidance given to me. Their constructive feedback and propensity for detail were catalysts to improve my work and ensured completion of work.

Thanks to the Commonwealth Scholarship Fund for the opportunity to study at Victoria University of Wellington, an opportunity that has empowered me to make meaningful contributions to my country's development. Special thanks to the NZAid Team that supported me throughout my journey in New Zealand.

Special thanks to the faculty and staff at the Graduate School of Nursing, Midwifery and Health, as well as Victoria University of Wellington for the support I received and opportunities I was given during my time as student. I am also grateful to my colleagues, friends, and Student Learning Support Services who took time out of their busy schedule to proofread portions or all of my scripts. I must also acknowledge the valuable contribution of the personnel from the Ministry of Health, Jamaica who provided well needed data by email throughout the course of my study and I am eternally grateful to all the participants without whose contribution this project would have been futile.

Finally, I would also like to acknowledge my family, students and friends who were always there to assist and provide support at some stage of my work. Thanks especially to my son Romaine who endured my absence from home for the entire period of study.

List of Abbreviations

A&E	Accident and Emergency Department
AIDS	Acquired Immune Deficiency Syndrome
CAT/CT	Computerised Axial Tomography
CARICOM	Caribbean Community
CHA	Community Health Aide
CHASE	Culture, Health, Arts, Sports and Education
CEO	Chief Executive Officer
CMO	Chief Medical Officer
CNO	Chief Nursing Officer
DR	Doctor
ECOSOC	Economic and Social Council
NP	Nurse Practitioner
GEASO	Government Employees Administrative Services Only
GDP	Gross Domestic Product
GNI	Gross National Income
HIV	Human Immuno-deficiency Virus
IDB	Inter-American Development Bank
ICN	International Council of Nurses
JADEP	Jamaica Drug for the Elderly Programme
JAMPRO	Jamaica Promotions Corporation
JIS	Jamaica Information Service
JSLC	Jamaica Survey of Living Conditions
KPH	Kingston Public Hospital

MDG/SDG	Millennium Development Goals/Sustainable Development Goal
MOH	Ministry of Health
MRI	Magnetic Resonance Imaging
NERHA	Northern Regional Health Authority
NGO	Non-Governmental Organisation
NHF	National Health Fund
NHS	National Health Services
NIS	National Insurance Scheme
ODA	Official Development Assistance
PAHO	Pan American Health Organisation
PATH	Programme of Advancement through Health and Education
PHC	Primary Health Care
PHI	Public Health Inspectors
PHN	Public Health Nurse
PIOJ	Planning Institute of Jamaica
RHA	Regional Health Authority
RN	Registered Nurse
SERHA	South East Regional Health Authority
SRHA	Southern Regional Health Authority
STATIN	Statistical Institute of Jamaica
STI	Sexually Transmitted Infections
UK	United Kingdom
UNICEF	United Nations International Children's Emergency Fund
USA	United States of America
USAID	United States Agency for International Development
UTI	Urinary Tract Infection
VEN	Vital Essential and Necessary
VJH	Victoria Jubilee Hospital
WHO	World Health Organisation
WRHA	Western Regional Health Authority

CHAPTER 1

Jamaica: A Perspective

INTRODUCTION

This monograph provides an introduction to Jamaica and its health system from a policy and structural perspective. It is intended to assist the readers to understand the historical and cultural climate within which the health system transitioned and currently operates, as well as highlighting significant developments and the current structure. The monograph includes a brief description of Jamaica as a country; the development and reform of the public health system from the 17th–21st centuries; health system funding from the 17th–21st centuries; and the delivery and utilisation of health services.

GEOGRAPHIC CHARACTERISTICS

Jamaica, a member of the Commonwealth of Nations, is the largest English speaking Caribbean island and the third largest country in the Caribbean Community (CARICOM). Jamaica has a land mass of approximately 10,991 square kilometres (km2) and lies 885 km south of Miami, Florida, in the United States of America (USA) and 145 km south of Cuba (Jamaica Promotion Corporation [JAMPRO], 2010). Administratively, Jamaica is divided into three counties: Cornwall, Middlesex, and Surrey, which are further subdivided into 14 parishes. The parishes within the counties are as

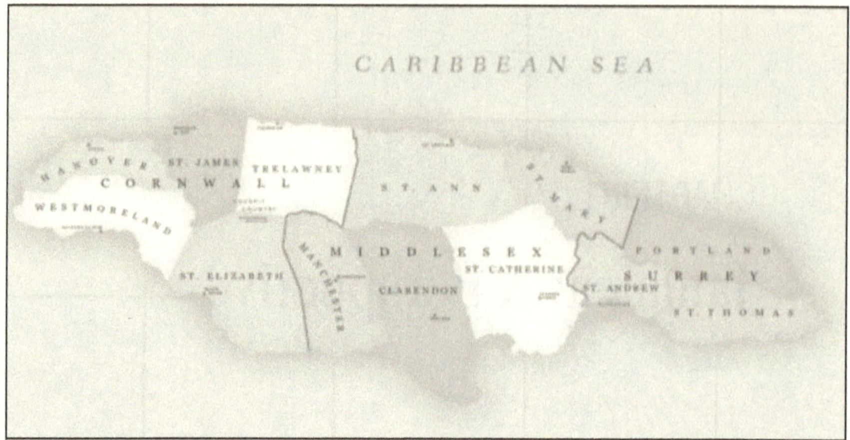

Figure 1. Map of Jamaica (Source: Pie a la Mode ©Action 4 Reel Filmworks, 2011). Reproduced with permission

folows: Cornwall – St James, Trelawny, Westmoreland, St Elizabeth and Hanover; Middlesex – Clarendon, Manchester, St Catherine, St Mary and St Ann, and Surrey – Kingston, St Andrew, Portland and St Thomas. Each parish has a capital and several districts. There are two major cities, Kingston, the capital, and Montego Bay, one of the main tourist resort areas (Figure 1) (Pan American Health Organisation/World Health Organisation [PAHO/WHO], 2007).

DEMOGRAPHIC CHARACTERISTICS

Jamaica had a population of 2,698,810 at the end of 2009 (Statistical Institute of Jamaica [STATIN], 2010) with a population growth rate of 0.2% over 2008 (Planning Institute of Jamaica [PIOJ], 2011). Jamaicans are predominantly of African descent – 97%, East Indian – 1.3%, European – 0.2%, Chinese – 0.2%, mixed - 0.7% and other – 0.6% (Jamaica Ethnic Group, 2009). In 2009, the age distribution comprised 0–14 years (27.4%, male 378,762/female 360,906), 15-64 years (64.1%, male 849,073/female 880,471) and 65 years and older (8.5%, male 101,506/female 128,091) (STATIN). Of note, is that the 15–64 age group is increasing and 65 years and older is the fastest growing group in proportion. Conversely, the 0–14 age group is declining. The ageing population may be a result of a reduction in fertility and mortality rates in addition to increased migration rates. The age profile has implications for the health sector both in terms of the development of programmes for the prevention and management of chronic non-communicable diseases, as well as adequate health financing for this group (MOH, 2009c).

In 2010, Jamaicans had a life expectancy of 74.13 years (STATIN, 2010), which compares well with global trends (UNDP, 2011; World Bank, 2011). The infant mortality rate was 16.7 deaths per 1,000 live births. The maternal mortality rate was 94.8 per 100,000 live births. The crude birth rate was 15.4, and the crude death rate was 6.0 per 1,000 population. The total fertility rate stood at 2.4 children per woman (STATIN). The infant and maternal mortality rates may have implications for Jamaica's achievement of global targets such as health-related Millennium Development Goals (MDG) (PIOJ & Ministry of Foreign Affairs and Foreign Trade [MFAFT], 2009).

Jamaica enjoys good health status generally (Watson Williams, 2008), has a good primary health care (PHC) track record and compares well internationally; for example, immunisation coverage in 2010 was at 95% whereas global coverage was 85.3% (PIOJ, 2011; World Bank, 2011).

POLITICAL CHARACTERISTICS

Jamaica is a former British colony. Having obtained its independence in 1962, the nation opted to remain within the British Commonwealth. The Queen is represented by a native Governor General, who is recommended by the Prime Minister. The Westminster Whitehall model of Parliamentary democracy is used with 'first past the post' general elections, which can only be called by the Prime Minister every five years. It has bicameral legislature; Cabinet governance; and Ministerial assignments (Jamaica Constitution 1962; MOH, 2009c; PAHO/WHO, 2007; WHO, 2010a).

There is an inextricable link between the diversity of the population and the country's history of Plantocracy, also called Slavocracy (a political system in which white landowners dominated the government) (Black, 2011). The Jamaican motto "Out of Many One People" aptly reflects its ethnic composition, as well as accentuating the unity embraced by the Jamaican people as they contribute to nation building (Jamaica Information Service [JIS], 2007). Consistent with international trends there is increased urbanisation in Jamaica. Half of the population reside in urban areas, especially in the Kingston Metropolitan Area. This essentially is a result of industrialisation (PAHO/WHO, 2007), which has encouraged people to move to urban areas in search of jobs and better quality of life.

SOCIAL AND HEALTH CHARACTERISTICS

Social indicators for Jamaica for 2006–2010 are shown in Table 1. Despite the fluctuating trends for some indicators it is important to note the achievements made over the years in the Human Development Index, literacy rates,

Table 1: Social Indicators for Jamaica 2006–2010

Indicators	Years				
	2006	2007	2008	2009	2010
Population	2,669,542	2,682,120	2,692,358	2,698810	2,705,800
Population growth (annual %)	0.5	0.5	0.4	0.2	0.3
Human Development Index	0.710	0.717	0.724	0.724	0.726
Enrolment in primary school ('000)	318.7	310.0	315.1	307.8	294.7
Literacy rate (%)	85.5	86.0	86.4	86.8	91.7
Labour Force (Total)	1,229,633	1,243,867	1,256,272	1,228,415	1,223,195
Unemployment rate (%)	10.3	9.8	10.6	11.4	12.4
Access to safe water	77.3	78.7	81.1	81.3	88.0

Source: PIOJ. (2011). Economic and Social Survey Jamaica 2010. Kingston, Jamaica: Author.; STATIN. (2010). *Demographic statistics 2009.* Kingston, Jamaica: Author; UNDP. (2011). (2011). *International Human Development Indicators.* Retrieved from http://hdrstats.undp.org/en/countries/profiles/JAM.html; World Bank. (2011). *World Development Indicators.* International Bank for Reconstruction and Development/ The World Bank, Washington D.C. Author.

and access to safe water. Enrolment in primary school has seen a minimal decline, which may be attributed to the decline in fertility rates. Another area of concern is the high unemployment rate, which has implications for the economy generally, and the health sector and the health of the nation by extension.

The nation is on track with targeted health-related MDG with successes in reducing absolute poverty, malnutrition and hunger. In addition, universal primary enrolment has been achieved. In 2009, gross enrolment in primary schools was 99.5% for children aged 3–11 years (PIOJ & STATIN, 2010); and progress is being made in providing safe drinking water and reducing the prevalence of HIV/AIDS *inter alia* (PIOJ, 2009). The estimated adult (15–49 age group) HIV prevalence rate was 1.7% in 2009, with approximately 21,000 Jamaicans of all ages living with the disease (United Nations International Children's Emergency Fund [UNICEF], 2010).

ECONOMIC CHARACTERISTICS

Despite perennial fiscal problems, Jamaica is currently classified as an upper middle-income country (World Bank, 2011). The economy has been negatively affected by servicing an external debt burden (4th highest debt-to-Gross Domestic Product (GDP) ratio in the world) (Economic and Social Council [ECOSOC], 2009) and, more recently, by contraction in the economy as a spin-off from the global recession, especially in revenue generated from remittances. To achieve some stability in the economy, the government renewed its relationship with the International Monetary Fund in 2010 (Johnston & Montecino, 2011). The country had a GDP per capita of US$5,133 in 2010 (Table 2).

Despite marginal increases in recurrent budgetary allocation, there has been a decline in capital budgetary allocation generally. For the financial year 2010/2011, an estimated $32.7 billion was allocated to the health sector, a 6.9% increase over the 2009/2010 financial year. Additional funding in the sum of $62.7 million was generated from new initiatives by the government, for example, the Jamaica/Cuban Eye Care Programme (PIOJ, 2011), introduced in 2005.

Table 2: Economic indicators for Jamaica 2006–2010

Indicators	Years				
	2006	2007	2008	2009	2010
GDP per capita (current $US)	4,616	4,949	4,994	4,615	5,133
GDP growth rate (%)	3.2	0.6	-1.7	-2.6	-0.6
Inflation, consumer prices (annual %)	8.6	9.3	22.0	9.6	12.6
External debt stocks (% GNI)	70.84	86.58	76.18	91.42	104.21
Net ODA received (% of GNI)	0.3	0.2	0.7	1.3	1.1

Source: PIOJ. (2011). *Economic and Social Survey Jamaica 2010.* Kingston, Jamaica: Author; World Bank. (2011). *World Development Indicators.* International Bank for Reconstruction and Development/ The World Bank, Washington D.C, USA: Author.

ENVIRONMENTAL CHARACTERISTICS

Jamaica is susceptible to frequent natural disasters such as hurricanes and storms, which, undoubtedly, affect its progress economically. Disruption in the agricultural sector from these phenomena over the years has resulted in a decline in exports of produce such as sugar, banana and coffee. However, through governmental assistance to improve the robustness in the sector, there was some growth in 2010. The growth was realised despite damage caused by Tropical Storm Nicole to crops and livestock amounting to $576.5 million (PIOJ, 2011). The environment portfolio falls within the ambit of the MOH and, as such, has implications for funding of the health sector.

INDIGENOUS PEOPLE AND THE SPANIARDS

Historically, the first inhabitants of Jamaica were the Tainos (also called Arawak Indians) from South America. Very little is documented about these natives because by the 18th century they were exterminated due to the

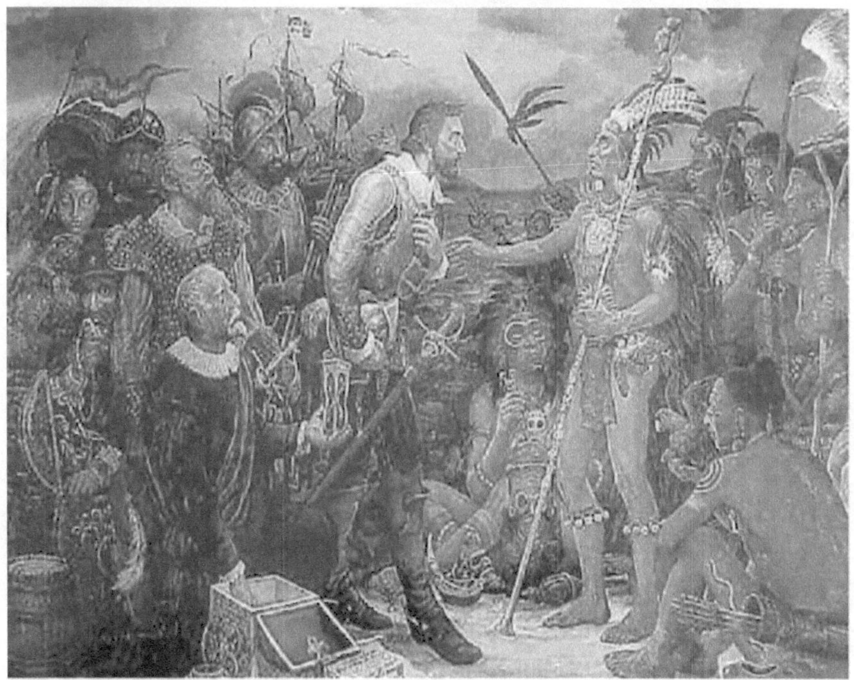

Arrival of the Spaniards in 1494

exploitation of the Spaniards and Europeans. Subsequent to the incursion of Christopher Columbus and Spanish convoys in 1494, mortality rates among natives increased exponentially. As a consequence of the high mortality rate among the natives there were fewer labourers to work on the plantations that were established by the Spaniards. Therefore, they resorted to African slave workers in 1517 (Black, 2011; Warner-Lewis, 2002). Mortality rates among the Tainos were so startling that "In 1598 the Governor of Jamaica Fernando Melgarejo was alarmed at the speed [with] which the Indian population was dwindling" (Black, p. 27). While many Indians died of the harsh treatment meted out to them by the Spaniards, others committed suicide or infanticide in order to escape the realities of slavery. Additionally, other Indians died as a result of infectious diseases brought into the country by the Europeans. Indians' farms were also destroyed by the Europeans' animals such as cattle and goats, leaving very little cultivated land for their survival. The decimation of the natives continued throughout the reign of the British, who conquered the Spaniards and occupied the country in 1655 (Robertson, 2002).

BRITISH SLAVOCRACY

Between the period 1655 and 1838 Jamaica was known for its Plantation System, mainly sugar plantations, which were first introduced by the Spaniards. Sugar production was an economically viable commodity at the time and Jamaica, a leading producer, had a reputation for producing quality sugar (Higman, 2005). To maintain this status, British estate owners expanded the slave trade and brought the enslaved in large numbers from Africa to sustain their plantations, which were villages equipped with all the facilities for the production and manufacturing of sugar. This essentially was the precursor to the widely-known slave trade to Jamaica (Black, 2011). After much resistance by estate owners, Jamaica achieved full emancipation in 1838 (Campbell, 2002), a process that commenced with the Abolition Act of 1833. This process was further strengthened by pockets of sustained activism against the inhumane treatment of slaves on the plantations. Notable activists included Granville Sharp, William Wilberforce and William Knibb.

Of note, however, is that estate owners were averse to ending slavery because "sugar was the crop that produced the greatest wealth and the best opportunities for long term financial success" (Higman, p. 18). This resulted in the introduction of the Apprenticeship system. Under this arrangement, ex-slaves were employed to work 40½ hours per week for the estate owners without compensation (Black). The Apprenticeship system was transitory

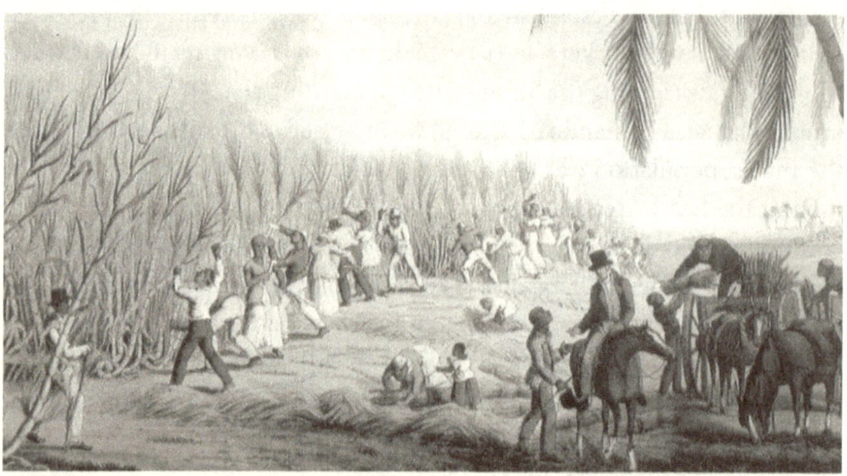

Enslaved Africans on a sugar plantation

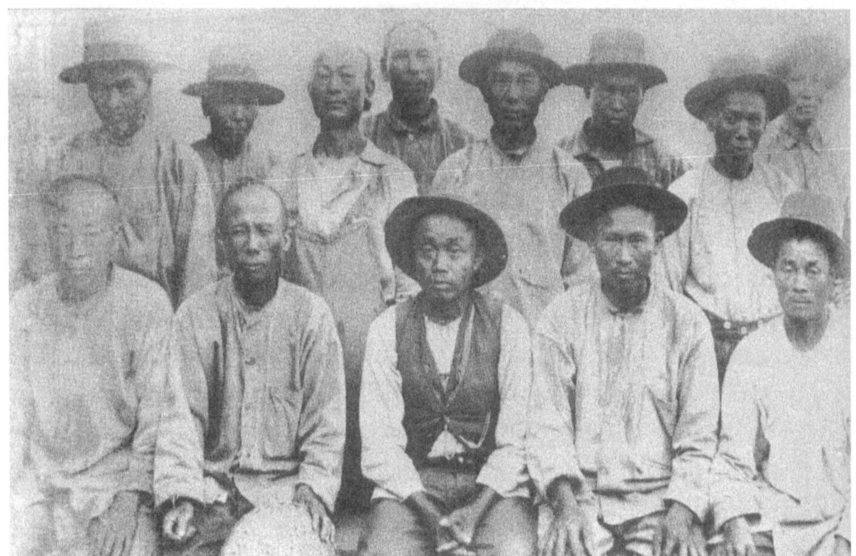

Chinese indentured workers

because reports of the brutal treatment of apprentices resulted in the passing of a resolution in England that signalled its end in 1838. Absentee estate owners had to seek labourers elsewhere (Black). For this reason, persons from India and China were brought to Jamaica as indentured or contract labourers to work on the plantations (Campbell, 2002).

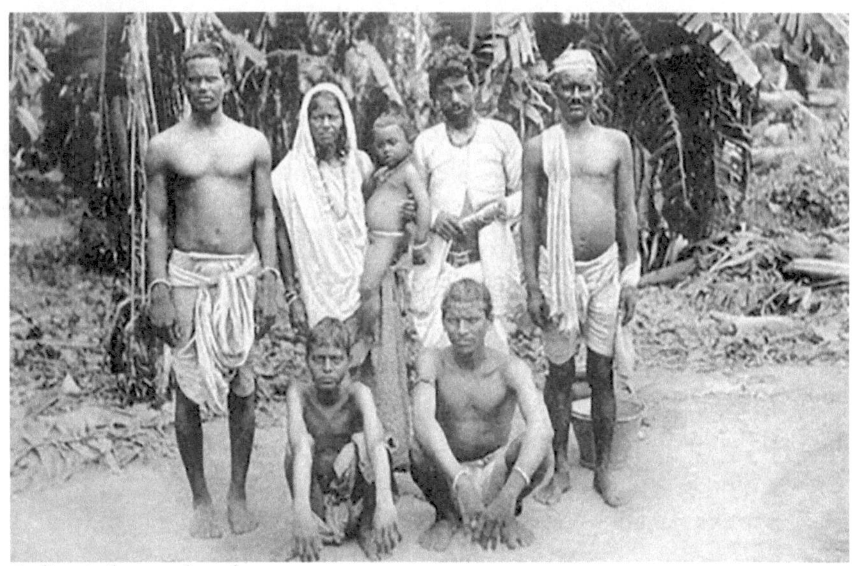

Indian indentured workers

OVERVIEW OF HEALTH CARE SYSTEM IN JAMAICA

Recent efforts by the Jamaican government to enhance access to health care were fast-tracked by data from the *Jamaica Survey of Living Conditions 2007*. The data revealed that approximately 50.3% of Jamaicans in the lower socioeconomic group were not accessing health care despite their illnesses (PIOJ & STATIN, 2008). The evidence indicated that the cost of services and socioeconomic status were determinants in individuals' ability to access health services.

Jamaica has a two-tiered health sector, which comprises both a public and private sector. This text focuses primarily on the public sector; however, a brief description of the private health sector will also be provided. Despite the dearth of literature on the private health sector in Jamaica, the available information suggests that it is utilised by individuals as an alternative to the public sector. The private sector is largely unregulated, and therefore has minimal obligatory responsibilities to the MOH (Health Sector Task Force, 2009). Both systems will be discussed further in this text.

Differences between the two systems are highlighted below. Delivery of public health care is provided by four Regional Health Authorities (RHAs) through a network of primary, secondary and tertiary health care facilities. The public health services are funded by an annual national budgetary allocation from the government, revenues collected from user fees, funds donated by international bilateral and multilateral development agencies (MOH, 2008a), and gifts. Table 3 shows the expenditure on health for the period 2006–2010. While the figures portray some volatility in funding over time, they also highlight the significant role played by out-of-pocket expenditures. For some users of the public health sector, health insurance is not a reality and, as such, many experience difficulty obtaining care when required, especially from private providers.

In contrast, private health care is available to consumers who can afford it. Private health care is provided by general practitioners and a network of institutions offering health services, mainly in the area of pharmaceuticals and diagnostic services. These private health facilities may be located within the 14 parishes and are not managed or regulated by the RHAs. Such services are funded by individuals through fees charged for services. Fees for services in the private sector usually exceed the charges for care in the public

Table 3: Health financing indicators in the Jamaican public health sector 2006–2010

Indicators	Year				
	2006	**2007**	**2008**	**2009**	**2010**
Total health expenditure (% GDP)	4.2	4.9	5.2	4.9	4.8
Per capita total health expenditure (current $US)	187	230	272	228	247
Public expenditure on health as a % of total expenditure on health	54.7	52.0	53.5	55.4	53.5
Out-of-pocket expenditure (% private expenditure on health)	63.7	71.0	71.0	71.0	71.0

Source: World Bank. (2011). *World Development Indicators.* International Bank for Reconstruction and Development/The World Bank, Washington D.C, USA: Author

sector. Users of the private health sector often hold health insurance (PIOJ & STATIN, 2008). Of note is that some public health institutions also provide privately-funded health services for those who require it.

Health insurance is provided mainly by private companies and has been used to offset the cost of health care in Jamaica. *The Jamaica Survey of Living Conditions 2007* revealed that more persons in the upper quintiles (where the statistical sample is divided into fifths, in which quintile 1 is the lowest and quintile 5 is the highest on the social status scale) have access to this arrangement in comparison to those who are of low socioeconomic status. This was more pronounced in the rural areas where health insurance coverage was lowest, albeit the group with a high percentage of individuals reporting illness but who did not seek health care (PIOJ & STATIN, 2008). The survey also found that increased health insurance coverage paralleled an increase in the number of individuals from the various quintiles (PIOJ & STATIN). These findings corroborated data from other studies (Flores et al., 1998; Hussey et al., 2007). Health insurance will be discussed in more detail later.

Choice of health care facility is sometimes based on individuals' perception of quality and efficient service delivery (Kiwanuka et al., 2008;

Nabyonga et al., 2005). Choice of facility, however, is not confined to these factors. Other factors influencing choice include distance from facility, transportation, diversity of the service or how technologically advanced the service is, operating hours, cost of the service, access to health insurance, preference, and severity of illness (MOH, 2008a).

Although consumers of health care in Jamaica have access to both public and private health care, data from *The Jamaica Survey of Living Conditions 2007* highlighted that, over time, there was an increase in the number of persons reporting illness and injury in all quintiles. Significantly, the findings showed that those in quintile 1 had a lower utilisation rate of the health system than those in the higher quintiles (PIOJ & STATIN, 2008). Despite the ability to choose, some consumers were challenged by issues relating to affordability and accessibility of care.

For this reason, policymakers are constantly monitoring the progress of health care and the quality of life of the nation's people through health indicators such as mortality rates and life expectancy (MOH, 2008a). In recent years, initiatives such as the Jamaica Drug for the Elderly Programme (JADEP), Programme of Advancement through Health and Education (PATH), the Culture, Health, Arts, Sports and Education (CHASE) Fund and the National Health Fund (NHF) have been implemented to improve access to health care services, especially pharmaceuticals. These initiatives will be discussed in more detail later.

Accessing health care, whether public or private, from both hospitals and health centres, involves a journey and patients can be either hindered or facilitated at varying stages. Persons facilitating the process include nurses, pharmacists, doctors and other health care providers. Noteworthy is that several categories of nurse facilitate the process at different stages of a patient's journey. Professional nurses in the secondary care settings include registered nurses (RNs) or staff nurses, ward managers and directors of nursing services, and in the PHC settings there are nurse/midwives, public health nurses (PHNs) and nurse practitioners (NPs). NPs attend to patients who are similar to the patients seen by doctors in both the secondary and PHC settings, while the PHNs focus on maternal and child health services. Nurses' roles are discussed further in this text.

Nominal fees used to be charged for health care services, especially in the PHC setting. These, however, were found to be one of the barriers to accessing health care in the public health sector. Geographic location was also identified as a barrier, especially for people living in the rural areas (PIOJ & STATIN, 2008). To meet the demand of this segment of the population, policymakers resorted to establishing new categories of health workers such as the NPs from as early as 1977 and expanding the role of others such as midwives in the 1970s (McCaw-Binns, Moody, & Standard, 1998).

The debate on user fees in the Jamaica public health system has been ongoing. As a result, on May 28, 2007 user fees were abolished for children under 18 years and an election promise was made by the incumbent government to abolish user fees in 2008 for all users of the public health system. The Minister of Health, in a statement validating the government's position on the abolition of user fees, mentioned the relationship between well-being and development (JIS, 2008), further reiterating the inextricable link between the growth of a nation and the health of its people. Subsequently, fees were removed for all users of public health facilities (hospitals, health centres, laboratories, diagnostic facilities, pharmacies) on April 1, 2008 (MOH, 2008b, 2008c).

This move was intended to indirectly improve access to health care services for the poor. The MOH in outlining the policy context noted that:

> The imperatives that informed the abolition of user fees policy are not unique to Jamaica and are as follows: (a) user fees policy has been shown to be regressive and a major impediment to access to health. *The Jamaica Survey of Living Conditions 2007* show that 50.8% of the poorest quintile who reported an illness did not seek health care because they could not afford so to do; (b) user fees have increased poverty because they reduce the disposable incomes of the poor and deplete their asset base; (c) user fees policy impacts negatively on utilisation resulting in deteriorating health outcomes, increasing morbidity and reduced life expectancy. (MOH, 2008b, p. 1)

The aims of the policy included eliminating impediments to access, creating an equitable health sector, reorienting PHC, relieving health staff of administrative tasks such as assessment of patients and collection of fees, and identifying suitable alternative financing and modes of service delivery (MOH, 2008b). Reports indicated a 125% increase in utilisation of some health facilities in the days following the removal of user fees (MOH, 2008d, 2009a).

CHAPTER 2

Development and Reform of the Jamaican Health System

In the absence of easily accessible archival material, a document prepared by the MOH Health Sector Task Force in 2007 was used to provide background on the history of the public health sector in this chapter. The Jamaican health system evolved over time and has its history embedded in the Plantation System. While there is limited documented evidence on the health services for the native people prior to the arrival of the Africans, reports implied that 'medicine men' treated sick Tainos and that folk medicine was often adopted for ailments (Hay Ho Sang, 1985). The following discussion highlights the form of health service delivery system in existence during the colonial period. The historical underpinning of the health system is one of oppression, inequity and mistrust. This has influenced political and social reforms, as well as the policy directives of the nation and the manner in which people respond to the processes over the years.

PLANTATION SYSTEM, 1658–1838

During this period, Jamaican society was pluralistic and greatly influenced by Plantocracy (Black, 2011). The health system, which dates back approximately two-and-a half centuries, was hierarchical in nature (Health Sector Task Force, 2007), providing quality services for the whites and substandard services for the blacks. A glance at the Plantation System reveals a health

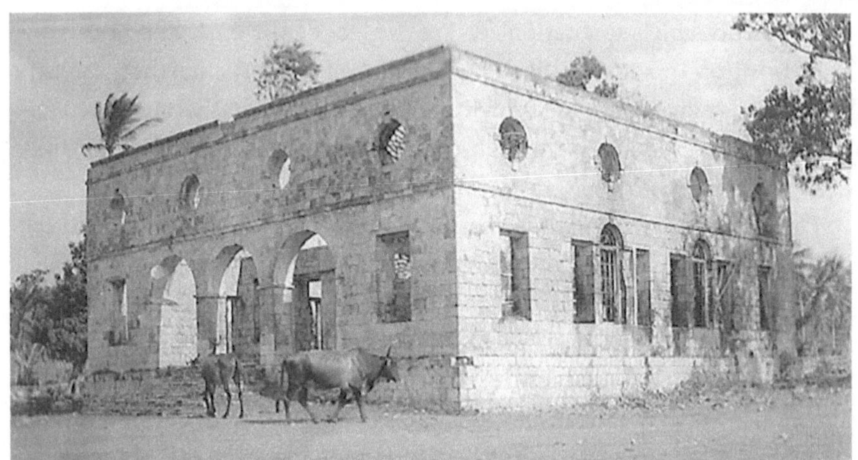

Enslaved hospital at Orange Valley, Trelawny, built in 1797

system in which health care for the enslaved was not a priority and inhumane treatment of the enslaved a daily occurrence. Epidemics among the enslaved were widespread, mainly because the attention estate owners gave to the health of the enslaved was negligible. Diseases affecting the slaves included yaws, dysentery, yellow fever, small pox, tuberculosis, and worm infestations. In addition to the epidemics, there were reports of high incidences of infant mortality rates, maltreatment, overwork and starvation among the enslaved (Health Sector Task Force; McCaw-Binns & Moody,

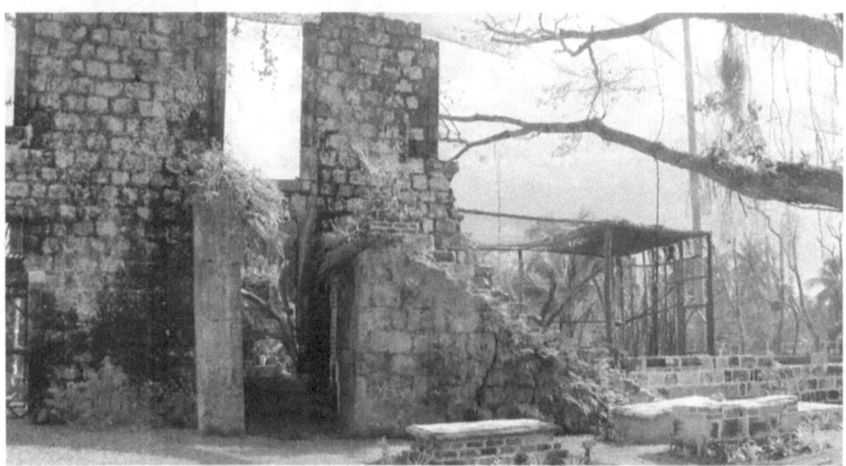

Ruins of enslaved hospital at Good Hope Plantation in Trelawny

2001). A possible explanation for the neglect of the enslaved' health was their position in society; they were treated as property. Furthermore, the death of a enslaved was not a challenge for estate owners, because a replacement could be obtained through the lucrative slave trade without much difficulty.

Despite lacking an organised structure, by 1774 the health system had military hospitals and a naval hospital in the main cities at which medical officers administered health services on a capitation basis (Golding as cited in McCaw-Binns & Moody, 2001). In 1776, the first public hospital, the Kingston Public Hospital (KPH), was established and served as a hospital, almshouse and asylum (Swaby, 2005). It provided health care exclusively for whites. Categories of health workers included medical officers, who had responsibility for demographics such as births and deaths, management of infectious diseases, and hygiene on the properties generally. They also delivered health care to the plantation owners, their families, and the house slaves. Although limited attention was given to the health needs of slaves, records indicated they were treated by doctors in hospitals known as "plantation hospitals" or "hot houses" (Black, 2011, p. 137). In contrast to the military hospitals, these facilities were sometimes managed by veterinarians (Health Sector Task Force, 2007). There were also nursing homes for those

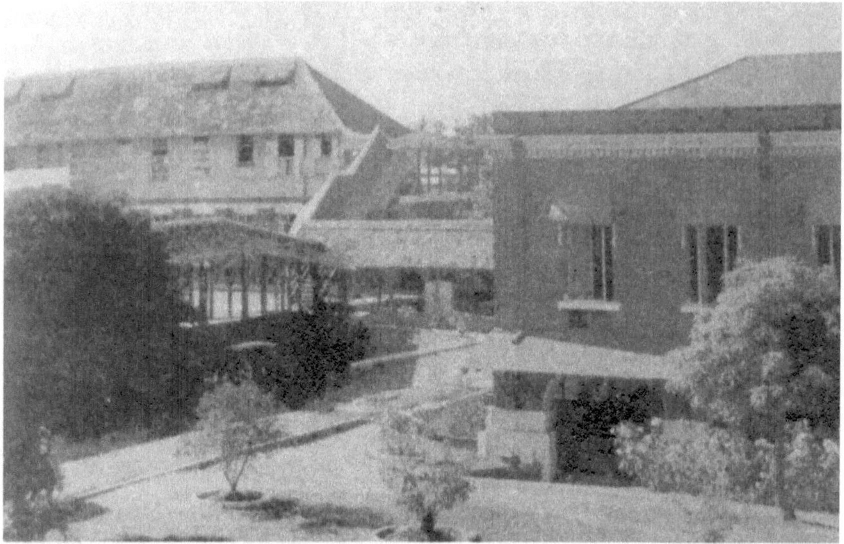

Kingston Public Hospital, 1946

who could pay for the services (Hay Ho Sang, 1985). In addition to medical officers, records make reference to other categories of health workers, namely "grandees", "wet nurses" and 'doctresses', who assisted with the care of the sick, and the pregnant and dying slaves (Swaby, p. 16). Nanas (untrained midwives) and nurses also delivered care to the sick (Hay Ho Sang). Golding, in identifying the category of staff in hospitals during this era, asserted that the staff included "one part-time physician, two apothecaries, a matron and five slaves" (as cited in McCaw-Binns & Moody, p. 7). They provided care to individuals who could not afford to pay for services.

Given the high mortality among slaves, poor health services and intolerable treatment meted out to them, anti-slavery movements raised consciousness regarding the evils of the system and, in 1792, the Consolidated Slave Act was enacted in Britain, giving slaves the right to improved health services (Health Sector Task Force, 2007). One of the articles of this Act dealt with the mandatory submission of reports by medical officers, regarding the number of deaths among slaves, as well as causes of death. These data had not been previously reported (Health Sector Task Force). Despite these arrangements, the inhumane treatment of slaves persisted. Poor living conditions, unacceptable health care and maltreatment of slaves were often a reality on the plantations for many more years.

EARLY EMANCIPATION, 1839–1846

After the abolition of slavery in 1838, extensive changes took place in the social system, which served as catalysts for change in the health system. Notable changes in the social system included movement of slaves away from the plantations, with only a few loyal slaves remaining, which led to the collapse of operations on the plantations (Health Sector Task Force, 2007). In 1846, the Sugar Equalisation Act was passed, further dismantling the plantation system. As a result, medical officers' incomes declined; therefore, they migrated to other countries such as England in search of employment (Health Sector Task Force; McCaw-Binns & Moody, 2001). These changes contributed to the deteriorating social and health conditions of the nation. The deteriorating conditions occurred because earnings from the plantations were non-existent and inadequate provision for ex-slaves

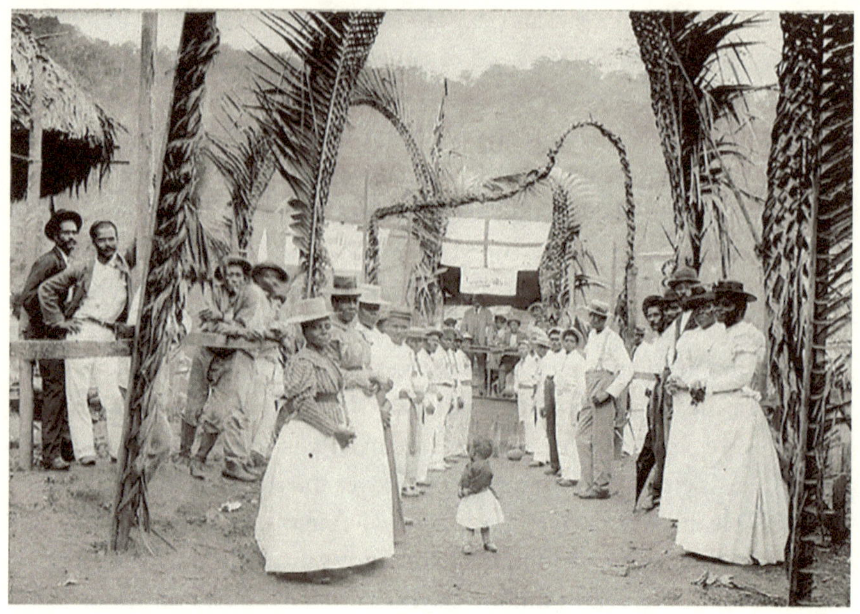

Emancipation Day, Jamaica

inevitably resulted in anarchy. Furthermore, the absence of medical officers in a poorly organised and ailing health system created an environment that was conducive to epidemics.

COLONIAL POST EMANCIPATION (CROWN COLONY PERIOD), 1847–1900

The demise of the Plantation system impacted negatively on the health and social systems of the nation in several ways and, as such, crises were inevitable. There were hardships, empty hospitals, migration of doctors, deteriorating health conditions and widespread epidemiological crises (McCaw-Binns & Moody, 2001). Epidemics affecting the country included typhoid fever (1853), cholera (1850 and 1852) and smallpox (1852). For these reasons, mortality and morbidity rates were high and all the parishes were affected. The death rate from cholera was "1 in every 13 of the population" (Black, 2011, p. 118).

Of note is that Mary Seacole, one of Jamaica's first nurses, began her nursing career in 1850 during the cholera outbreak (Black; Swaby, 2005). There

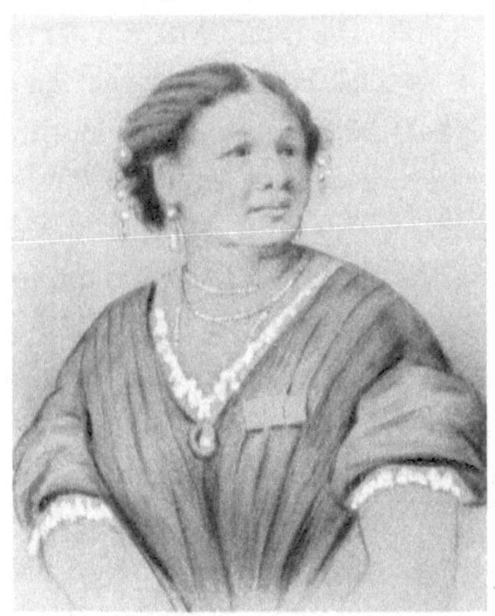

Mary Seacole

is a dearth of information on nurses training during this period of time. However, some training commenced as early as 1856 at the Lady Barkly Training Institution (Hay Ho Sang, 1985; Swaby). It was apparent that a link existed between the post-emancipation reduction in the number of medical officers and the increasing epidemiological crises (McCaw-Binns & Moody). A possible explanation is that no alternative provision was made for the health care of the free slaves generally (Black). Even though there was a lack of alternative health care and shortage of medical officers, the care of individuals affected with yellow fever and cholera was effectively administered by nurses, some of whom were known as "doctresses" at the time (Swaby, p. 16).

British governors continued to rule the country post-emancipation and in 1866 the reigning Governor, Edward John Eyre, replaced the constitution with a Crown Colony government. Under the Crown Colony, the governor formed the government and had sufficient power to make far-reaching changes to the social welfare of the nation (Black, 2011). Eyre became unpopular, and was later dismissed and recalled to England following a Royal Commission into the Morant Bay Rebellion of 1865. The rebellion which took place in Morant Bay, St Thomas, was the result of deteriorating social conditions in the nation. The commission revealed that Eyre's authority was a contributing factor to the rebellion. Eyre's successor, Governor Sir John Grant, was appointed the same year. Grant's work heralded in the new Jamaica, resulting in the development of organised social and health systems (Black).

Public Health Act and Boards of Health

As the years progressed, the improvements made by Grant reflected advancements in the health system. For example, in 1867, the Public Health

Law was enacted resulting in the establishment of the Island Medical Services or Central Board of Health (Health Sector Task Force, 2007; McCaw-Binns & Moody, 2001; Public Health Act, 1985). Parochial Boards of Health were subsequently instituted in all 14 parishes, through which the agenda of the Central Board of Health was implemented. The Parochial Boards had the task to create a link between health and the country's development, to quarantine and treat diseases, and to provide public health care, including safe water supplies, proper roads and communications (Black, 2011; Health Sector Task Force). The intention of this system was essentially to provide services to freed enslaved people and indentured labourers regardless of their income.

In addition to the establishment of the health boards, there was a proliferation of dispensaries (modern day health centres) in all 14 parishes. These facilities were hospital-outstations, offering health services in Kingston from as early as 1870 (Cover, 1995; McCaw-Binns & Moody, 2001). Information on the exact number and location of these facilities is not available. Some plantation hospitals which were closed following emancipation and migration of medical officers were reopened with the aim of making health services more accessible to the greater populace. Additionally, District Medical Officers were deployed to 40 medical districts that were established among the 14 parishes in 1874 (Cover; Health Sector Task Force, 2007), and in 1887 the first Lying-In facility, the Victoria Jubilee hospital (VJH) was established in response to a maternal mortality rate in excess of 600/100,000 births. It was so named because construction occurred in the year that Queen Victoria celebrated her Golden Jubilee (McCaw-Binns, 2008).

THE NATIONAL HEALTH SERVICES (NHS) SYSTEM, 1901–1938

By the turn of the century, there was a myriad of noticeable developments in the health system. Firstly, there was rationing of hospital services as a result of overcrowding. This was evident in the revocation of funding allocated for health services to the poor in 1904. Subsequently, funding of health services was replaced with a ticket system in 1933–1934 in an attempt to ensure accessibility (Cover, 1995). Secondly, more hospitals were built across the country between 1916 and 1926, which ultimately resulted in the 'hospitalisation' of the health system. Despite the colossal improvement in public health, there was still discrepancy between the support for community-based and hospital-based health services. Support for hospital-based services was evident in the increased workforce assigned to hospitals versus the limited number of District Medical Officers (DMOs) assigned to community health services. Moreover, the budgetary support for community health services was inadequate. This created a need to forge greater links between the two levels of health services in order to provide a more equitable and accessible health service delivery system. Thirdly, the number of DMOs, private practitioners and other health practitioners increased during this era (Health Sector Task Force, 2007).

Appointment of Commissions

An equally significant feature of this period was the appointment of landmark commissions to investigate the health and social conditions of the nation. Widespread riots against ineffective governance and deteriorating social conditions were often catalysts for the appointment of commissions of inquiry (Health Sector Task Force, 2007). Essentially, riots were mechanisms adopted by ex-slaves to attract the attention of the Colonial Government to their situation and have it act in line with the interests of the masses. Key commissions during this period included the Rockefeller Foundation Commission and the Moyne Commission (McCaw-Binns & Moody, 2001).

At the end of World War I, the Rockefeller Foundation Commission (1918–1932) was appointed to investigate the deteriorating public health conditions of the nation. The work of the Commission was significant and involved the investigation of epidemics such as hookworm (1918), tuberculosis (1927), malaria (1928) and yaws (1932) (McCaw-Binns & Moody, 2001). As a result of the recommendations contained in the Rockefeller Commission's report, the Bureau of Health Education was established in 1927 and a new cadre of staff, PHNs and public health inspectors (PHIs) (sanitary inspectors), was introduced. The roles of the new health personnel included management of communicable diseases. Nurses were involved in delivering social services, while PHIs managed the home and community environments (McCaw-Binns & Moody). Sensitising the population about preventive measures was an equally important role for both nurses and PHIs.

Further, support from the Rockefeller Commission resulted in the provision of fellowships and grants for the training of additional health personnel and the establishment of health facilities. Facilities established under the support of the Commission included a tuberculosis clinic and tuberculosis sanatorium. Consequently, through the implementation of the recommendations of the Rockefeller Commission there was noticeable improvement in the control of communicable diseases and importantly the eradication of some diseases such as malaria by 1961 (McCaw-Binns & Moody, 2001).

Concerns were again raised in 1938, when there were widespread riots, and infectious diseases were among the five leading causes of death (McCaw-Binns & Moody, 2001; Watson Williams, 2008). These conditions were drivers for the appointment of the Moyne Commission (1938–1939) to investigate conditions in the nation and the West Indies generally. Through the Commission's recommendations, epidemiological, social and political strategies were implemented, which resulted in a reduction in mortality and morbidity rates, as well as improved quality of life for the nation's people.

Training facilities for health personnel were also established and included the Training Station for Sanitary Inspectors and Health Visitors (renamed as the West Indies School of Public Health in 1957), now known as the University of Technology, Jamaica, School of Public Health. The School enrolled its first entrants in 1944 (McCaw-Binns & Moody). Further recommendations by the Moyne Commission included reorganisation of the health services and allocation of a minimum 10.0% of the national budget to health services (West India Royal Commission, 1945). The Commission also highlighted the "relationship between health and poverty, housing, public health . . . community development and adequate funding of community health services" (Health Task Force, 2007, pp. 29–30).

Impact of natural disaster

While the deteriorating social conditions could not be attributed to any one factor, one possible reason for the minimal improvement in social and health services during the early 20th century was the impact of natural disasters on the island. Such catastrophes shift the interest of authorities from social and health needs to restoring the affected areas (McCaw-Binns & Moody, 2001). One notable event was the earthquake of 1907 in which the country was devastated (Black, 2011). It is not uncommon for disasters to erase the gains made in the health and social system, further plunging the country into a state that requires the government to seek external assistance. The impact of the aforementioned earthquake overwhelmed hospitals and the number of deaths was high. External assistance in the form of medical supplies and health personnel was obtained from the USA (Black). In the face of the ongoing situations, health services continued to deteriorate, with the greatest impact on the poor and vulnerable.

PRE-INDEPENDENCE – SELF GOVERNMENT PERIOD, 1939–1962

Social and economic development continued throughout this period; however, due to the effects of World War II there was delay in timely implementation of the recommendations of the Moyne Commission. Despite the delay, health services continued to expand and additional commissions of inquiry were appointed including the Irvine Committee in 1944.

The Irvine Committee

This Committee was appointed to investigate the contentious health conditions as part of a larger investigation being undertaken in the British colonies at the time. The recommendations of the Committee were catalysts for the establishment of the University College Hospital of the West Indies (now the University Hospital of the West Indies) and the training of medical doctors, which was initiated in 1948. The training of doctors took precedence because there was sufficient evidence to suggest health conditions in the nation were deteriorating (McCaw-Binns & Moody, 2001).

Crown colony and independence

Amidst the challenges to social and health conditions in the country, the political change process continued. One such change involved embracing self-government in exchange for Crown Colony status. This was achieved under the provision of a new constitution in 1944. Jamaica now had a legislature that included a House of Representatives and Legislative Council. Additionally, the new constitution empowered Jamaicans with additional rights under Adult Suffrage. Jamaicans 21 years and over became eligible to vote during elections (Black, 2011; Health Sector Task Force, 2007). Undoubtedly, this gave voice to the poor in matters of national importance such as issues surrounding health and social conditions.

Additional changes in the health system during this era included the amalgamation of the Medical Department into the Ministry of Health (MOH) in 1955. Accordingly, a leadership structure emerged which included a Minister of Health, a Permanent Secretary, a Chief Medical Officer (CMO), Principal Nursing Officers and Assistant Nursing Officers for secondary and primary services (Health Sector Task Force, 2007).

Another significant milestone achieved by Jamaica in 1962 was independence from British rule. This signalled not only a change in the political structure but also in the health system. The country was now fully self-governing and the Ministry of Health's focus was on hospital services. The hospital-based services offered were influenced by international standards and, as such, were similar to the American hospital-centred model of health system (Health Sector Task Force, 2007). This ultimately resulted in the 'hospitalisation' of the health system to the detriment of Primary Health Care (PHC).

THE POST-INDEPENDENCE PERIOD, 1963–1971

Expansion in health infrastructure and services

In the Post-Independence period, additional hospitals were built with the assistance of funding from the World Bank. One such institution was the Cornwall Regional Hospital, a Type A Regional hospital in St James. This institution was fraught with design faults, which resulted in some departments being abandoned. Possible reasons for the glitches included cultural differences, in that the facility was fitted with an infrastructure similar to European hospital design. The design provided for warmth in the winter season, whereas Jamaica is a tropical country. The lack of consultation with main stakeholders such as nurses was also problematic.

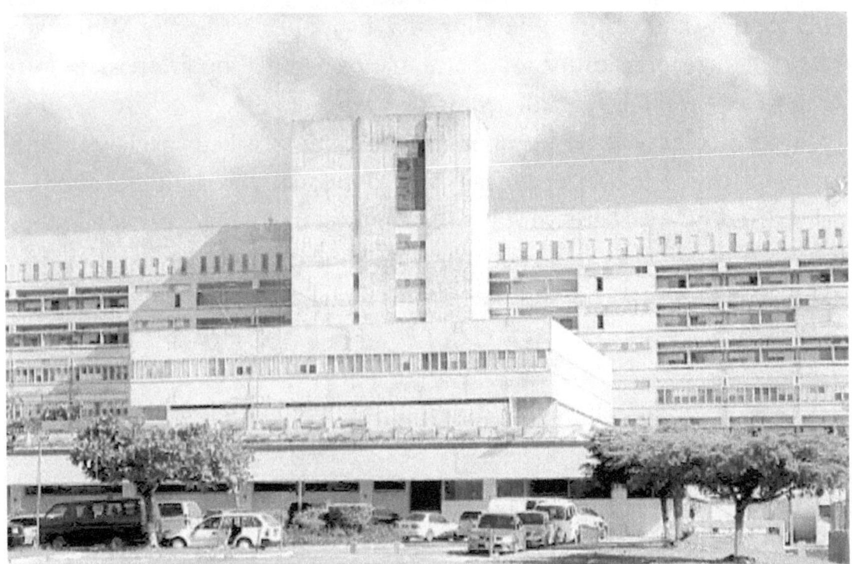

Cornwall-Regional Hospital, Montego Bay

Notwithstanding setbacks, advancement in the social conditions continued and there were observable demographic changes such as population explosion. According to the Health Sector Task Force (2007),

> Jamaica entered the stage of a demographic transition. Improvement in health status of the population resulted in lower death rates and greater birth rates with high dependency ratios and demonstrated the inability of the economy to sustain the rapid rate of population increase (p. 35).

As a result of the increase in birth rates, a Family Planning Service was established in 1967 under the umbrella of the National Family Planning Board, which was supported by the World Bank. In addition to the development in family planning, there were attempts to privatise the system. For example, private beds were introduced into the public health system as a means of encouraging privatisation.

Reform in the governance of the health system

Occurring in the post-emancipation period was a greater separation between Central and Local Boards of Health, whereby the Ministry of

Finance now had responsibility for MOH supplies, while the Ministry of Works had responsibility for maintenance, even though artisans were assigned to hospitals (Health Sector Task Force, 2007).

Fundamental changes occurring at this time included special arrangements instituted, by way of a means test, for people who could not afford to pay for health care. Moreover, little or no budgetary assistance was allocated to health centres that functioned in an unplanned manner. A possible explanation for this practice was the strong focus placed on hospital-based services.

Development in the health workforce

There was also inaugural training of community health aides (CHAs) in 1967. Their role as members of the health team included working in the community in areas such as maternal and child health, health education and promotion, and disease prevention (McCaw-Binns & Moody, 2001). Additionally, there was the introduction of dental nurses and dental assistants in 1970 (McCaw-Binns & Moody). They functioned predominantly in the PHC settings and were instrumental in offering school dental services.

Despite the training of new cadre of health personnel, one should not be oblivious to the effects of the 1962 Cold War political tensions on Jamaica, which resulted in mass migration of health personnel, similar to the exodus in 1846. As a consequence, a bilateral accord was forged in the 1970s between Jamaica and Cuba for the supply of health workers, among other arrangements, in order to maintain a stable health system (Health Sector Task Force, 2007).

MODERNISATION OF THE HEALTH SYSTEM, 1972–1989

Throughout the 20th century, robust policy initiations further impacted on the development of the health sector. For example, in 1972 the Environment Control Portfolio was placed under the MOH. This move by the government was lauded by some stakeholders, who felt this would impact positively on the development of the nation (Health Sector Task Force, 2007).

New nomenclature, management and fees system in hospitals

A national policy initiative implemented at the local level included new nomenclature for hospitals. The categories were determined by virtue of the

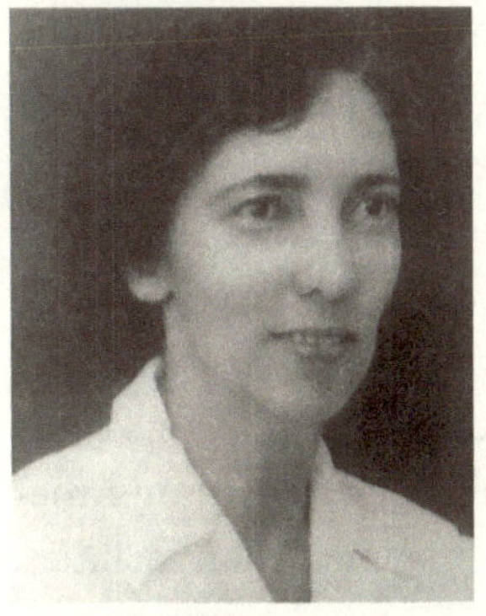

Gertude Swaby

services offered and comprised Types A, B, C and D. These categories will be discussed in more detail later. Additionally, hospital boards were established in 1972 and, hospitals were now governed by a Board of Management (Health Sector Task Force, 2007). Subsequent to the establishment of hospital boards, user fees were removed for public health services. This policy change formed part of the ongoing reform and hinged on the premise that the revenue generated from user fees was inadequate for an equitable and sustainable health system (Health Sector Task Force).

Green Paper 1974

In 1974 a Green Paper "*The Health of the Nation*" was ratified in parliament. This was a significant event in that the implementation of the Green Paper's recommendations vastly influenced the public health system. Some of the recommendations included introducing charges for drugs, establishing a Central Planning and Evaluation unit to oversee the amalgamation of secondary and PHC services, offering PHC services in health centres, locating health centres to meet the needs of the population within their boundaries, managing pharmaceutical services by engaging advanced techniques and expertise, and retaining staff by adopting measures such as better working conditions, remuneration commensurate with work done and making post-graduate training facilities available for health workers, *inter alia* (Health Sector Task Force, 2007).

New roles and categories of staff

In order to achieve acceptable coverage for maternal and child health services, the role of the midwife was expanded in the 1970s. This move was to provide quality maternal and child health services to the underserved population in the rural areas, as well as to relieve the PHNs of some tasks. PHNs were now able to focus on specialty-oriented tasks. This initiative resulted in increased antenatal visits island-wide (McCaw-Binns & Moody, 2001).

Training of health workers continued in this era. Another category, NPs, commenced training and joined the workforce in 1977. They were deployed to the health system on completion of extensive training. NPs function mainly in the PHC setting with a focus on curative services (McCaw-Binns & Moody, 2001) and deliver specialist health services in various settings. They work in parallel with the medical officer in health centres. NPs' roles were expanded in order to be responsive to the needs of people, especially in certain geographic areas, for example, rural and poorer communities (Safriet, 1992). In addition to providing services in some urban facilities, NPs in Jamaica offer services to individuals living in rural communities. The elderly and the poor benefit the most.

Other important events in the era

Five events occurred during this period. The first main event occurred between 1976 and 1977 and involved some level of organisational reform in the public health system, including the integration of Central and Local Boards of Health. The aim was to reduce the fragmentation in delivery of health services, which had contributed to the lack of proper mechanisms to manage and monitor the transformation taking place. One factor that may have been responsible for this situation was the notion of shared management responsibilities in which the MOH had responsibility for hospital services, while Local Government had responsibility for Parish Health Services (Health Sector Task Force, 2007). Secondly, a National Formulary was established between 1977 and 1980 to strengthen the management and delivery of pharmaceutical services in the country (Health Sector Task Force).

Thirdly, PHC research commenced and was conducted through PHC units in Jamaica. This served as the launching pad for 'The Primary Health Care: Jamaican Perspective' policy that was formulated in 1978. The success of this work influenced the appointment of Jamaicans to serve on the Drafting Committee of the Alma Ata Declaration of 1978 (Health Sector Task

Force, 2007). The fourth event was the introduction of compulsory immunisation in 1978 for all Jamaican children in order to prevent childhood immunisable diseases such as tuberculosis, poliomyelitis, diphtheria, tetanus and pertussis. To enforce this law, proof of immunisation became mandatory prior to entry into school and parents had a legal obligation to ensure their children were immunised. As a result of this policy, the rate of immunisable diseases was significantly reduced (Health Sector Task Force).

The fifth event was reforms in the hospital system. The aims of these reforms were to achieve a greater level of efficiency in service delivery, as well as to modernise the secondary and tertiary level services. Some hospitals involved in the reform process included the Bellevue Hospital, a psychiatric institution, which changed to a "decentralised therapeutic hospital" with over 1000 beds (Health Sector Task Force, 2007, p. 59) and the May Pen Hospital, where a new hospital was constructed. Construction of the facility was achieved with the assistance of the Inter-American Development Bank (IDB).

The impact of structural adjustment on the health system

The effects of the country's involvement with the International Monetary Fund (IMF) must not be ignored, since some reform processes were a direct result of Structural Adjustment in 1979 under the IMF. This resulted in austerity measures, which impacted on the delivery of health services. There was drastic budgetary adjustment (one third reduction) between 1982 and 1987 (Watson Williams, 2008). As an outcome there was a mass migration of health workers and a reduction in the training of some groups such as CHAs and nurses. Additionally, the rationing of the health services resulted in the closure of some training institutions and health facilities. Institutions affected included the Cornwall School of Nursing, The West Indies School of Public Health, and Type D hospitals, as well as some health centres (Health Sector Task Force, 2007). In addition to creating a gap in the health sector's human resources, the quality of services declined and shortages of equipment and supplies was a daily problem (Watson Williams). These issues increased the country's level of susceptibility to health conditions that had either been under control or successfully eradicated. The robustness of the PHC services declined and immunisation rates plummeted in the aftermath of the IMF interventions. Epidemics such as poliomyelitis re-emerged in the 1980s, which had serious implications for the tourist industry, one of the country's main sources of income (Health Sector Task Force).

MODERN HEALTH REFORM, 1990–2008

Regional Health Authorities

In addition to unremitting discussion about the country's PHC system, more health reforms occurred during the latter part of the 20th century. These reforms included regional integration of the management of primary and secondary health care under one umbrella. Integration of the systems was achieved through decentralisation and the enactment of the National Health Services Act in 1997 (National Health Services Act, 1997). Under the provisions of this Act, four semi-autonomous Regional Health Authorities (RHAs) were established. The RHAs, which are defined by geographical boundaries, are of varying sizes and have overarching responsibility for a number of parishes (Figure 2). It is important to note that the parishes assigned to the RHAs differ somewhat from county parishes mentioned earlier. The four RHAs comprise:

1. **The North East Regional Health Authority (NERHA).** NERHA is mainly rural and has a land mass of 2,637.1 km². It consists of three parishes, Portland, St Mary and St Ann, and in 2010 served a population of 371,900 (13.7% of the total population). NERHA is the smallest region with four hospitals, three health departments (a health department is located in each parish, is the administrative arm for PHC, is responsible and accountable for supplies such as vaccines for the parish and houses the office of the Medical Officer of Health) and 74 health centres (NERHA, 2009; Planning Institute of Jamaica [PIOJ], 2011; Ward & Grant, 2005).

2. **The Southern Regional Health Authority (SRHA).** SRHA is mainly rural and has a land mass of 3,238.8 km². It has three parishes, Clarendon, Manchester and St Elizabeth, and served a population of 591,500 (21.9% of total population) in 2010. The health facilities in this region include five hospitals, three health departments and 73 health centres (PIOJ, 2011; SRHA, 2011; Ward & Grant, 2005).

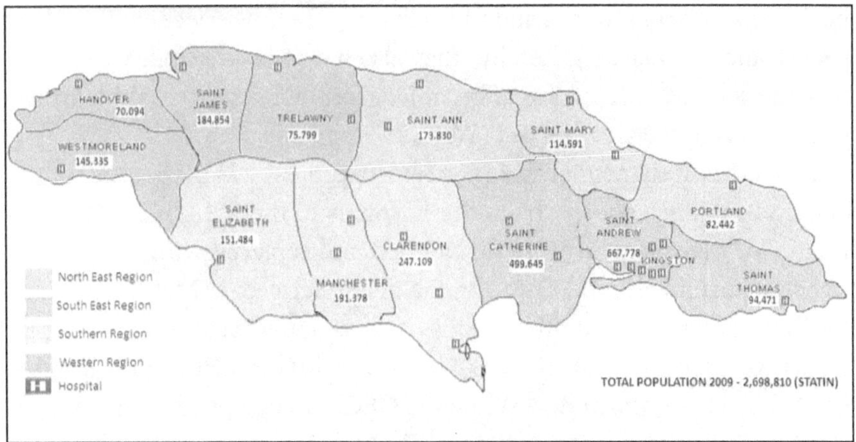

Figure 2. Hospitals and population by parish in the health regions (Source: Auditor General's Department, Jamaica, 2011). Reproduced with permission.

3. ***Western Regional Health Authority (WRHA).*** WRHA is mainly rural and has four parishes, Trelawny, St James, Hanover and Westmoreland. It has a land mass of 2,726.9 km² and served a population of 477,300 (17.6% of total population) in 2010. It has four hospitals, four health departments and 78 health centres (PIOJ, 2011; Ward & Grant, 2005; WRHA, 2009).

4. ***South East Regional Health Authority (SERHA).*** SERHA is mainly urban and has three parishes, Kingston and St Andrew, St Catherine and St Thomas. The region served a population of 1,265,100 (46.7% of the total population) in 2010 and has a land mass of 2,387.7km². It is the largest RHA and provides health services through a network of 10 hospitals, three health departments and 88 health centres (PIOJ, 2011; SERHA, 2010; Ward & Grant, 2005).

Structure and functions of the RHAs

RHAs are decentralised bodies with three overarching roles: policymaking, programme formulation, and programme execution (Health Sector Task Force, 2007). Policymaking is, however, not a primary role but rather a function of the MOH. Subsumed under these three roles are the RHAs' mandate to manage the allotted budgetary support, human resources, health related programmes and the delivery of health services within their geographic boundaries generally. They also have a responsibility to ensure that the services offered are affordable, acceptable and accessible to the populations in the areas served (Ward & Grant, 2005).

A significant element of this 1997 reform process was the transfer of the decision-making capacity from the hospitals to the RHAs. The Hospital Boards of Management were dismantled and replaced with a reporting structure that involves the Director of Nursing Services or Matron, the Senior Medical Officer, and other heads of departments reporting to a Chief Executive Officer (CEO). The CEO in turn reports to a Health Committee headed by an administrator. While the CEOs are equipped with management skills, there have been criticisms about their lack of nursing and medical knowledge that some believe is required to effectively oversee a hospital (Health Sector Task Force, 2007).

The move to regionalisation was based on the need to achieve greater efficiency, effectiveness and accountability in the delivery of health care and to reduce the concentration of power at the head office (Health Sector Task Force, 2007). Given the agenda prior to regionalisation, this element of the reform process resulted in devolution of power from the head office to the RHAs. Furthermore, the intention was to relieve the MOH of some of its functions in order to achieve a greater focus on the policy process, monitoring functions, and standards and regulations (Figure. 3) (Health Sector

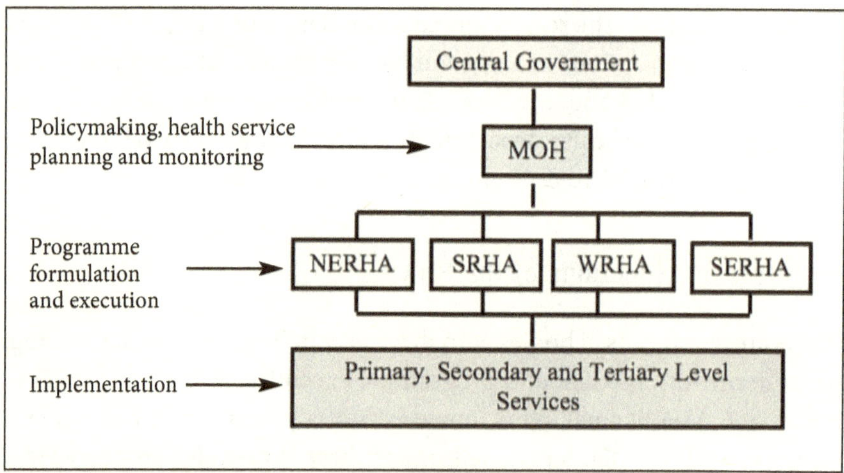

Figure 3. Structure and function of the public health sector

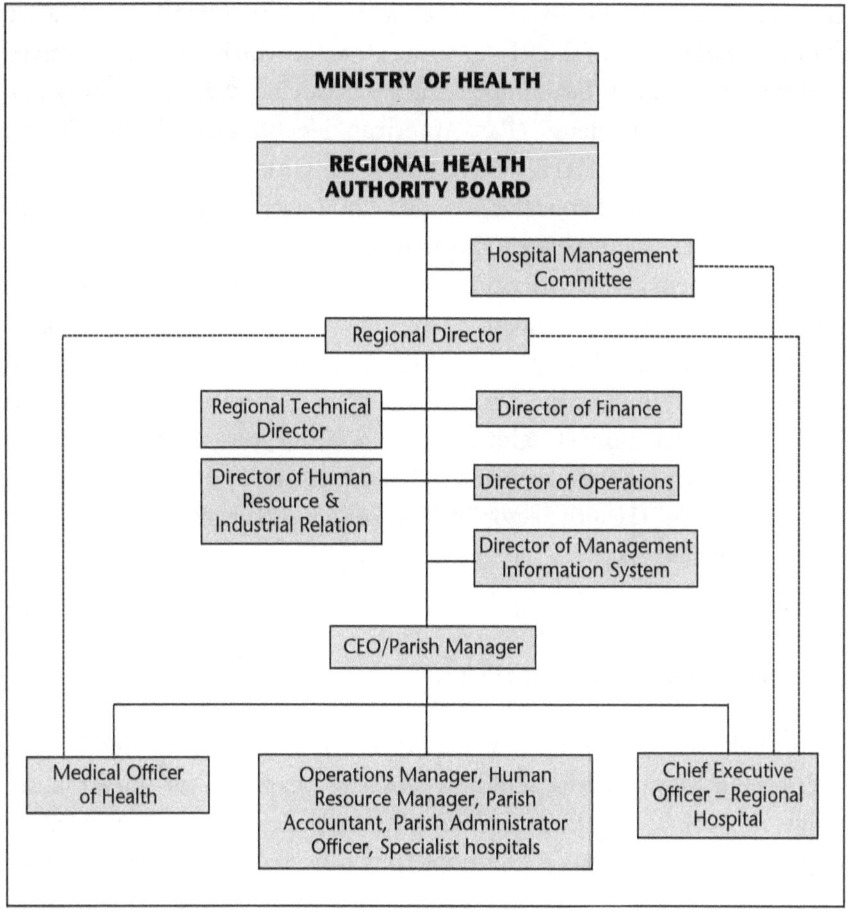

Figure 4. Structure of the Regional Health Authorities, Jamaica

Task Force). The RHAs' management structure comprises a Board to which the Regional Director reports. Additionally, the Directors report to the Regional Directors (Figure 4). The Boards are appointed by the Minister of Health, making each RHA accountable to the minister.

Evaluation of the RHAs

The RHAs have been providing health services for the nation since their inception in 1997, but not without the scrutiny of stakeholders and the population generally. While the intention of the reform was to improve efficiency, it is important to note that concerns have periodically been raised about the operations of the RHAs. Some areas for which they have received disapproval included "health planning, service delivery, accountability, and community involvement" (Pan-American Health Organisation/World Health Organisation [PAHO/WHO], 2007, p. 459).

Additional areas of concern included "moderate successes in cost-containment [and] negative effects shown in areas of personnel capacity, financial management and organisational capacity" (PAHO/WHO, p. 459). As a result of widespread discontent, a five-member Health Sector Task Force was appointed by the MOH in 2007 to investigate the RHAs' functions and contribution to the health sector, with a view to modernising the public health sector generally (Health Sector Task Force, 2007). The findings of the Task Force have been reported in the document "*A Healthy Jamaica in a Healthy World*" (Health Sector Task Force) but still await implementation by the policymakers.

REFORM OF THE PUBLIC HEALTH SERVICES IN 2007 & 2008

Reform of the health services in the 21st century included the abolition of user fees in May, 2007 for children under 18 years and for the Jamaican public in April 2008. The intentions of these policy interventions were to improve access to health care for poor Jamaicans; reduce inequity in accessing health services; reorient the public health system to reflect a primary care focus; enhance staff efficiency by providing the right skill mix for service delivery; and find suitable financing and service delivery mechanisms (MOH, 2008a). Under this new policy a number of health services were now free to users of the public health system.

To finance the latter policy, which was projected to lose $1.7m (approximately 12.0% of the health expenditure) by abolishing user fees, central government injected $3.85m to offset the health budget for 2008/2009 and meet the projected 30.0% increase in patient load (MOH, 2008a). Generally the Ministry of Finance & Planning earmarked $100m to fund the preparatory phase of the policy. This sum was disbursed to the RHAs incrementally and was to be used for infrastructural improvement; purchasing materials, supplies and equipment; and provision of transportation for staff, patients and supplies for efficient service delivery (MOH).

For effective policy implementation, strategies were adopted to address the perennial staff shortages. To respond to the projected increases in patient load, RHAs were advised to recruit and employ personnel such as nurses, doctors, pharmacists, and CHAs on a sessional or temporary basis; redeploy some staff; and employ public/private partnerships to acquire services such as medical and diagnostic (MOH, 2008a).

SUMMARY

It is apparent that the Jamaican social and health systems have been through a number of developmental stages, each resulting in reform. From the arrival of the Europeans to the gaining of independence, each stage has been influenced by social, economic and political occurrences locally and globally. The transformation of the country included graduating from colonial governance to self-governance; from an era with limited emphasis on human rights to one in which human rights are entrenched in its constitution; from an *ad hoc* health system to one that is more structured and formalised; from a society, in which health services were hierarchical with provision for select few, to universal health care, despite some inequity remaining in the system. Even though there was no real sense of stability, reforms have resulted in significant improvements in the social and health situations of the nation amidst stagnation in the economy.

CHAPTER 3

Financing The Public Health System

COLONIAL PERIOD AND CHARGES FOR HEALTH SERVICES

Information about funding of the public health system from the 17th–21st centuries is not well documented. Reports suggest that, during the colonial period, financing of the health system was mainly through, albeit negligible, budgetary allocation (Health Sector Task Force, 2007). Medical officers were paid a fixed fee per person to ensure wellness on the plantations (McCaw-Binns & Moody, 2001). Additionally, medical officers who had responsibility for the health care of estate owners and their households could charge a fee for services provided. While there was no formal fee structure, fees were reportedly charged according to the patient's earnings. This was achieved through a means test, which was first introduced in 1867.

In addition to the aforementioned, special arrangements were in place for the provision of free health services to indigents, the constabulary, prisoners and persons living in homes for the poor. A ticket system was also introduced in 1904, which made health services more accessible to the general populace (Health Sector Task Force; Cover, 1995). The ticket system was based on income of the patients (Table 4). There was limited change to this until the 1970s.

REFORM IN USER FEES SYSTEM

As alluded to earlier, fees were abolished for hospital services in the 1970s; however, limited information is available regarding the success of the policy

Table 4: Ticket payment system for outpatients

Income per week (shilling)	Charges
Family member earning = up to 16/-	Free
Family member earning = 20/-	Free
Family member earning = over 16/-to 35/-	1/6
Family member earning = over 35/-to 70/-	2/6

Source: Cover, W.A. (1995). *Handbook of Jamaica 1955. Ministry of Communications and Work. Kingston, Jamaica: Government Printing Office.*

change. User fees were, however, revised, reintroduced and increased in 1984, 1993, 1999 and 2005 (Barnett, Lalta, & Bailey, 2010; Lewis, 1993). A fundamental reason for the introduction of user fees was to generate revenue in the public health system. Revenue raised from the fees, however, was minimal, and some individuals cited out-of-pocket payment as having an adverse impact on access to health services (Planning Institute of Jamaica/Statistical Institute [PIOJ & STATIN], 2008). Moreover, the exemption process was considered demeaning by some individuals from the lower socioeconomic group. This compounded the problem of access; therefore, successive governments have proposed the abolition of user fees in order to improve access to health services.

The fee payment system was regarded as oppressive for some users, especially the poor, who did not utilise the services although there was a need (PIOJ & STATIN, 2008). For this reason, on May 28, 2007 user fees were abolished for children under the age of 18 years, and on April 1, 2008 for services in the public health system generally. Under this new arrangement, health services at the 23 public hospitals and over 313 health centres were provided without charges to the users. According to the MOH (2008a), the free services included but were not limited to:

registration, doctor's examination, hospital stay, diagnostic services (x-rays and laboratory tests of various kinds), drugs, physiotherapy, surgeries, family planning, immunisation, antenatal care, renal dialysis, drugs for chemotherapy, radiation therapy, certain high cost diagnostic services such as MRI [Magnetic Resonance Imaging] [and] certain high cost appliances. (p. 2)

Fees were retained by the public health system for several services. These included fees paid by private patients (persons with insurance and non-residents); fees for morgue services except for specific cases; medical examinations and reports obtained from PHC for business use; food handlers' fees; and medications and drugs for international travel (MOH).

JAMAICA AND OTHER CARIBBEAN COUNTRIES' EXPERIENCE WITH USER FEES IN THE 20TH CENTURY

In the 1990s, it was found that the Jamaican public health system was under-financed. As a result, the system was ailing from the reduced number of qualified staff, unavailability of pharmaceuticals, decreases in the quantity and quality of care provided, and dissatisfaction among workers and the wider populace. These challenges resulted in the introduction of a more extensive use of user fees for public health services. Revenue generated was to be utilised to boost expenditure on primary and secondary care services. The belief was that user fees would not adversely affect access to care or util-isation of the public health services. In addition, it was felt that revenues from user fees would be utilised to support management and overcome some of the challenges such as staff and drug shortages, and staff and patient dissatisfaction (Shepard, 1993).

Exemption policy

Caribbean countries such as St Kitts, St Lucia, St Vincent and the Grenadines, Dominica and Grenada also resorted to user fees to improve access to basic public health services. Each of these countries had exemptions for those who could not pay. In Jamaica, to enforce the exemption policy whereby people who could not afford out-of-pocket payments received services at no charge or at a subsidised rate, assessment officers were trained and deployed to the public health facilities. This arrangement was often disregarded by health facilities, especially for preventive services (Gordon-Strachan et al., 2010). The ineffective exemption process affected some individuals' ability to access health care, mainly due to their inability to pay out-of-pocket. One factor contributing to the ineffectiveness of the exemption policy was that users were often "afraid of being embarrassed" by assessment officers and health personnel for not being able to pay. This practice negatively affected the success of the policy (Gordon-Strachan et al., p. 147).

Van Doorslaer and Wagstaff measured horizontal equity (where people with equal need utilise the same amount of health care) in utilisation patterns in Jamaica through the application of a comparative econometric test on the Jamaica Survey of Living Conditions 1989. They found that utilisation of curative and preventive services in the public health system favoured the rich despite the poor having a greater demand (as cited in Gordon-Strachan et al., 2010). This further highlighted the ineffective exemption mechanism, which clearly did not protect the poor from the adverse effects of out-of-pocket payment for health care.

Studies in the Jamaican context on the effects of user fees on utilisation were varied and inconclusive in some cases. For example, Lewis and Parker (1991) found that revenue generated from user fees increased significantly for the period they studied; however, they offered no conclusion regarding the impact on utilisation patterns (as cited in Gordon-Strachan et al., 2010). Additionally, Shepard (1993) examined the impact of user fees in the public health system and found that hospital revenue increased annually following the introduction of user fees. There was, however, an inverse relationship with utilisation, as the utilisation trend of public facilities declined over the period studied. The decline was attributed to the quality of the services provided and not the increase in user fees.

Bailey, Wynter, Jackson and Lee (1994) examined the effect of user fees on access to family planning services at a quasi-health facility. Fees for this service were introduced in the facility in 1993. The study found that utilisation decreased by 28% between 1992 and 1993, and the decline was more pronounced among new users and users of injectable contraceptives. The authors concluded that users were unwilling to pay for a service that had previously been free. Equally, Alleyne (2010), in examining the impact of user fees on health costs and health burden among patients with diabetes and hypertension, found that user fees had a negative impact on health-seeking behaviour among Jamaicans. Individuals were found to reduce health-related costs by employing practices such as delaying or not seeking care when ill, purchasing only a portion of their prescribed medications, and using home remedies.

User fees were also found to have negative effects on the elderly. Evidence revealed that, despite the JADEP, the elderly who often required treatment for co-morbidities were unable to meet not only the costs for services, but also indirect costs for transportation, especially in rural areas. Elderly persons who were unable to access services in the primary preventive services often resorted to home remedies to manage their health conditions (Gordon-Strachan et al., 2010).

OTHER FUNDING INITIATIVES

Other funding initiatives by the government included public-private partnerships, which have contributed significantly to the public health system and initiatives such as the Jamaica Drug for the Elderly Programme (JADEP); the Culture, Health, Arts, Sports and Education (CHASE) Fund and the National Health Fund (NHF). The JADEP was established as part of the reform process in 1996. Under this programme, all Jamaicans aged 60 and older benefit from subsidised drugs for 10 chronic diseases including hypertension and diabetes. A JADEP membership card enables beneficiaries to access pharmaceuticals at reduced costs at participating public and private pharmacies (NHF, 2008).

The CHASE Fund of 2002 assists with financing of the public health system. It "receives, distributes, administers and manages monetary contributions from the lottery industry" (CHASE, 2008, para. 1), a percentage of which contributes to national development. The funds are allocated as follows: Sports Development (40.0%); Early Childhood Education (25.0%), Health (20.0%), and Arts and Culture (15.0%) (CHASE).

The NHF, a statutory body, was established in 2003. The fund is generated from "20.0% of special consumption tax charged on tobacco products; 5.0% of special consumption tax collected; and (0.5%) of annual earnings up to $500,000 paid by employee and employer, collected by the NIS" (NHF, 2008, para. 6). It provides additional funding for the health sector by subsidising the cost of drugs and providing support for the training of health workers, as well as providing assistance for the implementation of health-related programmes and infrastructural improvement.

The NHF is the conduit through which patients benefit from National Health Insurance-type services, which constitute a component of the health reform process (PAHO/WHO, 2007) as envisioned in the Green Paper of 1997 (Barrett & Lalta, 2004). The NHF embraced universal coverage for Jamaicans and its main objective is to improve the standard of services in the public health system by assisting individuals and institutions to better manage chronic diseases. NHF offers individual and institutional benefits. Approximately 50.0% of funds support individual benefits, while institutional benefits are available under two arrangements: one deals with health promotion, and the other with health support (Barrett & Lalta).

Beneficiaries access 1300 pharmaceutical services at both private (80.0%) and public (20.0%) facilities with the NHF card, which is also used to monitor individuals' use of services. The facilities are reimbursed on a weekly basis through a managed-fee-for-service arrangement (NHF, 2008). Of note is that a co-payment is required from the NHF beneficiaries. People pay the difference between the NHF remuneration and the price charged by the provider (NHF): "This serves as an incentive to be more deliberate in choosing where one gets a prescription filled" (Barrett & Lalta, p. 29).

DIVESTMENT OF HEALTH SERVICES

The divestment of some services in the health sector must not be discounted, because it constituted a part of the reform process in the 1990s. Through this mechanism, external resources were mobilised to foster efficiency and sustainability in the public health sector, further reducing health institutions' recurrent expenses. Among the health services divested were training of health personnel, dietary services, janitorial services and pharmaceuticals services (Figueroa, 2001; Shepard, Anthony, McNaught, & Davis, 1998).

BUDGETARY ALLOCATION

The Ministry of Finance has overarching control of the budgetary allocation to the MOH at the central level, which is further distributed to RHAs for service delivery (Health Task Force, 2007, 2009; PIOJ, 2011). Budgetary allocation to the RHAs is based mainly on the population served. RHAs are autonomous and independently allocate funds to the health facilities. Currently, the thrust is to reorient PHC and, as such, much budgetary support is given to curative services (PIOJ). RHAs may also adopt creative means to generate additional budgetary support for the programmes and services they offer.

In addition to the budgetary allocation from the Government of Jamaica, health funding is obtained through health insurance and gifts and donations from non-governmental (NGO) and international development partners such as the NHF, the Global Fund, United States Agency for Development (USAID), Inter-American Development Bank (IDB), The United Nations International Children's Fund (UNICEF), and PAHO/WHO. Generally, the support from these organisations included financing, maintenance, provision of health personnel and training (MOH, 2008b). Approximately 4.0–5.5% of Jamaica's national budget is spent on health services, which is considerably below the recommended proportion of 10.0–15.0% (Planning Institute of Jamaica & Ministry of Foreign Affairs and Foreign Trade [PIOJ & MFAFT], 2009). This limited funding is further compounded by the reality that Jamaica is now classified as an upper middle income country and no longer qualifies for assistance from some donor organisations.

HEALTH INSURANCE

Health insurance improves access to health care (PIOJ & STATIN, 2008) and, according to Gertler and Sturm (1997), may be a suitable mechanism to alleviate the financial pressure on the public health sector. A dual health insurance system exists in Jamaica: the British National Health Service model in the public sector, under which individuals obtain care at nominal cost, and the private health insurance model that provides coverage for 10.0% of the population (Health Sector Task Force, 2009). Individuals may have either private or government health insurance coverage. In contrast to public health insurance, private health insurance is largely unregulated (Health Sector Task Force) and obtained individually or cooperatively through an organisation. Health insurance may be obtained by self-employed and informal workers; however, it is mainly available to government and private company employees. The unemployed are usually excluded (Bourne, 2009).

The government's health insurance schemes are collaborative arrangements with private insurance companies. One example is the health insurance coverage for government employees, the Government Employees Administrative Services Only (GEASO) health care programme administered by Sagicor Life Jamaica. Under this arrangement, public sector workers are eligible for health insurance that is funded jointly by the government and the employees. The government makes a monthly contribution of 80.0%, while employees contribute 20.0%. There is also a Pensioners' Plan for retirees who are not eligible for individual or group coverage, and NI GOLD (National Insurance GOLD) for pensioners in the National Insurance Scheme (NIS). These arrangements allow pensioners continued access to health care benefits (Sagicor Life Jamaica, 2012).

Health insurance companies work collaboratively with participating health care providers, namely hospitals, pharmacies, private doctors, dentists, laboratories and eye care specialists to meet the health care needs of the insured. Services covered under the health insurance schemes include hospitalisation, outpatient care, surgical procedures, doctors' hospital visits, doctors' home visits, dental services, prescription drugs, diagnostic services and consultation fees (Sagicor Life Jamaica).

Individuals who hold health insurance have easier access to health services in both the public and private health sectors, since it "lowers treatment cost of illnesses . . . [and] lowers the psychosocial stressor on income, and [on] the family's wellbeing" (Bourne, 2009, p. 197). Individuals also have easier access to more expensive medications, diagnostic investigations and medical procedures. *The Jamaica Survey of Living Conditions 2009* reported that more people in metropolitan areas had higher health insurance coverage compared to those in rural areas. The report also revealed that most persons with insurance had private coverage. Despite an increase in the number of persons with health insurance coverage in the poorest quintiles (Quintile 1 & Quintile 2) in 2009, this group still had the lowest health insurance coverage generally (PIOJ & STATIN, 2010).

CHAPTER 4

Health Service Delivery and Utilisation of The Health Care System

Jamaica operates a health system in which approximately 95.0% of health services are offered by public health facilities, while the private sector provides the remaining 5.0%. The formal relationship between the private and public sectors is, however, negligible, despite the new thrust under the 2008 health sector reform process to forge and strengthen public-private partnerships in areas such as secondary care, and diagnostic and pharmaceutical services (Health Sector Task Force, 2009; Watson Williams, 2008). Among the providers of private health services are eight private secondary level facilities and over 2000 doctors working in urban and rural areas. Additionally, the private sector provides outpatient and PHC services, pharmaceuticals, health insurance and financing. The health services offered are usually more technologically-advanced than those offered in the public sector and include advanced services such as Computer Axial Tomography (CAT) scans, Magnetic Resonance Imaging (MRI), and specialised laser and cardiac surgeries among other cutting edge surgical procedures (Health Sector Task Force).

Despite being largely unregulated, the private health sector is accountable to the MOH, which has overarching responsibility for health. Moreover, the private health sector is required to adhere to the laws governing health practice in the country, for example, the Public Health Act.

The private sector is not without its share of challenges. For example, there is a perennial problem of a lack of resources for hospitalised patients and an inability to attract people from all socioeconomic backgrounds to utilise the services offered. This is often due to individuals' inability to afford the services in the absence of health insurance coverage. Policymakers, however, have attempted to alleviate the problems by providing tax relief for the providers of private health services and offering subsidised public health services to private patients. Of note is that information regarding the financing and performance of the private sector is not readily available (Health Sector Task Force, 2009).

HEALTH SERVICE DELIVERY

The public health system, the evolution of which was discussed earlier in this chapter, is regulated by the MOH and services are delivered by the RHAs through a network of 23 hospitals and over 313 health centres (Table 5). The services provided by the institutions may be at the primary, secondary, or tertiary level. Primary level services are located in the community at health centres or community hospitals, secondary level services in hospitals,

Table 5: Network of service delivery facilities 2010

Regional Health Authorities	Parishes	Population (%)	Facilities	
			Health Centres	Hospitals
North East	Portland, St Mary, St Ann	371,900 (13.7)	74	4
Southern	St Elizabeth, Manchester, Clarendon	591,500 (21.9)	73	5
Western	Trelawny, St James, Hanover, Westmoreland	477,300 (17.6)	78	4
South East	Kingston, St Andrew, St Thomas, St Catherine	1,265,100 (46.7)	88	10
Total		2,705,800	313	23

Source: Planning Institute of Jamaica (2011). *Economic and Social Survey Jamaica 2010.* Kingston, Jamaica: Author.

and tertiary level services at Type A public hospitals (e.g. Kingston Public Hospital, Cornwall Regional Hospital). Tertiary level institutions are also referred to as regional or teaching hospitals (PIOJ, 2011).

Types of hospitals

Type A hospitals are located mainly in major cities and deliver tertiary level services. They receive referrals from Types B and C hospitals. Type B hospitals are also located mainly in urban locales and are the referral institutions for Type C hospitals. Type C hospitals are usually located in rural communities and deliver general inpatient and outpatient services (Table 6) (SRHA, 2011; Ward & Grant, 2005).

Table 6: Classification of hospitals

Classification	Description
Type A	• Multi-disciplinary institutions offering secondary and tertiary care. • Final referral points for secondary and tertiary services.
Type B	• Situated in the large urban centres. • Provide inpatient and outpatient services. • Offer services in the following specialties – general medicine, general surgery, obstetrics and gynaecology, paediatrics and anaesthetics. • Offer x-ray and laboratory services to hospital patients, primary care and private sector locally.
Type C	• Basic district hospitals which interface with the primary care. • Offer inpatient and outpatient services. • Services offer include general medicine, surgery, maternity care paediatrics. • Offer basic x-ray and laboratory services to hospital patients, primary care and private sector locally. • Have a specialist surgeon for emergency surgical services.
Type D	• Closed under the structural adjustment programme.

Source: Southern Regional Health Authority, 2011

Types of Health Centres

Similarly, health centres are classified as Type I – Type V based on the type and level of services, as well as the population served. Type I health centres provide services in maternal and child health including immunisation, family planning, nutrition, and health education. Health personnel at these facilities include a registered midwife (RM) and at least two CHAs. The population served should be a maximum of 4000.

Type II centres provide services that are similar to but more advanced than the Type I facilities. Additional health personnel at Type II facilities include NPs, PHNs, staff nurses, doctors, PHIs and pharmacists. The population served should be approximately 12,000 (SRHA, 2011).

Type III health centres have a similar staff complement to Type II and serve a population of approximately 20,000. Services offered by Type III health centres include curative, maternal and child health, family planning, immunisation, nutrition, dental, environmental health, treatment of Sexually Transmitted Infections (STIs), contact investigation, pharmacy, mental health, counselling, and child guidance.

Type IV health centres are usually administrative departments with service delivery is at the parish level. These facilities are mainly located on a

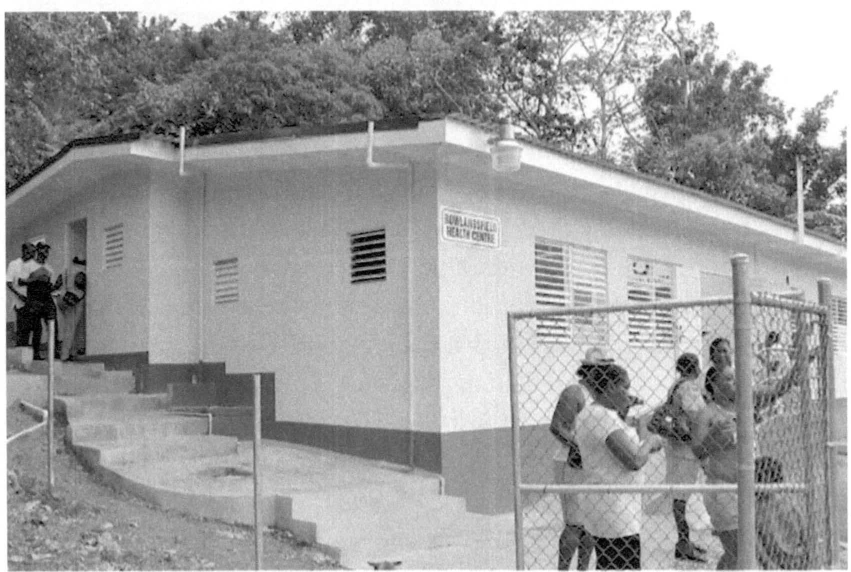

A rural Health Centre

hospital compound for easier access to diagnostic services. Type IV health centres offer the same services as Types I-III centres with the addition of mental health, Sexually Transmission Infection/Human Immunodeficiency Virus (STI/HIV) and dental services *inter alia*. Other categories of staff such as social workers, contact investigators and nutritionists may be found in these facilities.

Type V health centres are known as comprehensive health centres and provide all the services offered at the above-mentioned facilities. They are usually found in main cities (SRHA, 2011). Additionally, there are satellite stations among the PHC facilities (Health Sector Task Force, 2007). They offer services that parallel those of Type I health centres. These satellite stations are health centre outstations, which lack a physical structure.

Staffing for health facilities

Staffing of secondary care and PHC facilities is achieved through full-time and part-time employment. The RHAs employ various categories of staff mostly on a full time basis; however, some employees work part time. Individuals may opt to have dual employment status, whereby they work full time in one facility, usually a public facility, and on a part time basis in private facilities, and in exceptional cases they may have two part time jobs. For this reason, it is not uncommon to have health personnel who are employed simultaneously by both the private and public health sectors.

The main categories of health personnel employed in secondary care facilities include the director of nursing services or matron who has administrative responsibility for nursing services, medical doctors (including specialists), RNs (including specialists), RMs, enrolled assistant nurses, patient care assistants / ward assistants, emergency response technicians, PHNs (some hospitals), NPs (some hospitals), physiotherapists, speech therapists, radiographers, medical technologists, pharmacists, electrocardiogram technicians, nutritionists, and dieticians (Figure 5). Heads of department in secondary care facilities report to a CEO. Services offered at hospitals vary according to the type of facilities. For example a cardiology unit may not be found in a Type C hospital.

The medical officer of health has leadership of the PHC services and works in collaboration with PHNs, NPs and other health practitioners (Fig-

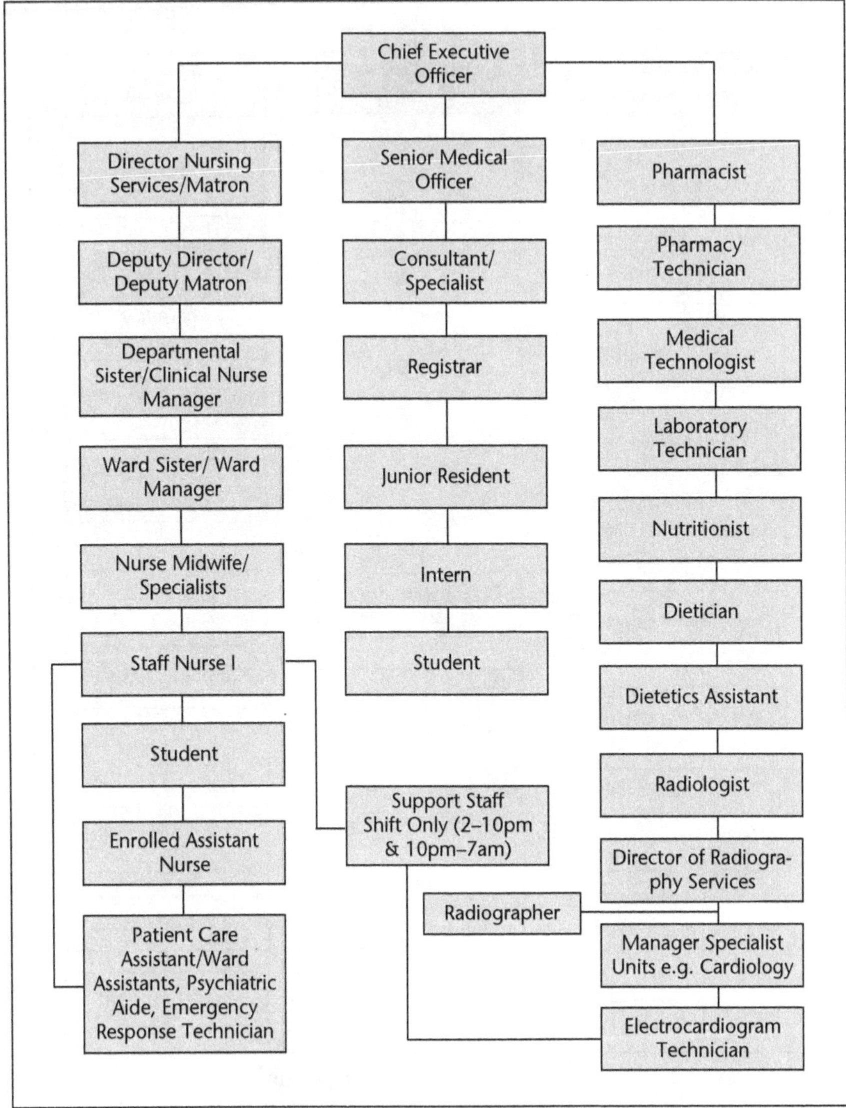

Figure 5. Typical structure of a Public Health hospital

ure 6). The requirement for employment in the health sector involves health personnel meeting the eligibility criteria for practice, which entail obtaining the necessary training from accredited institutions, registration, and licensure from the respective regulatory bodies.

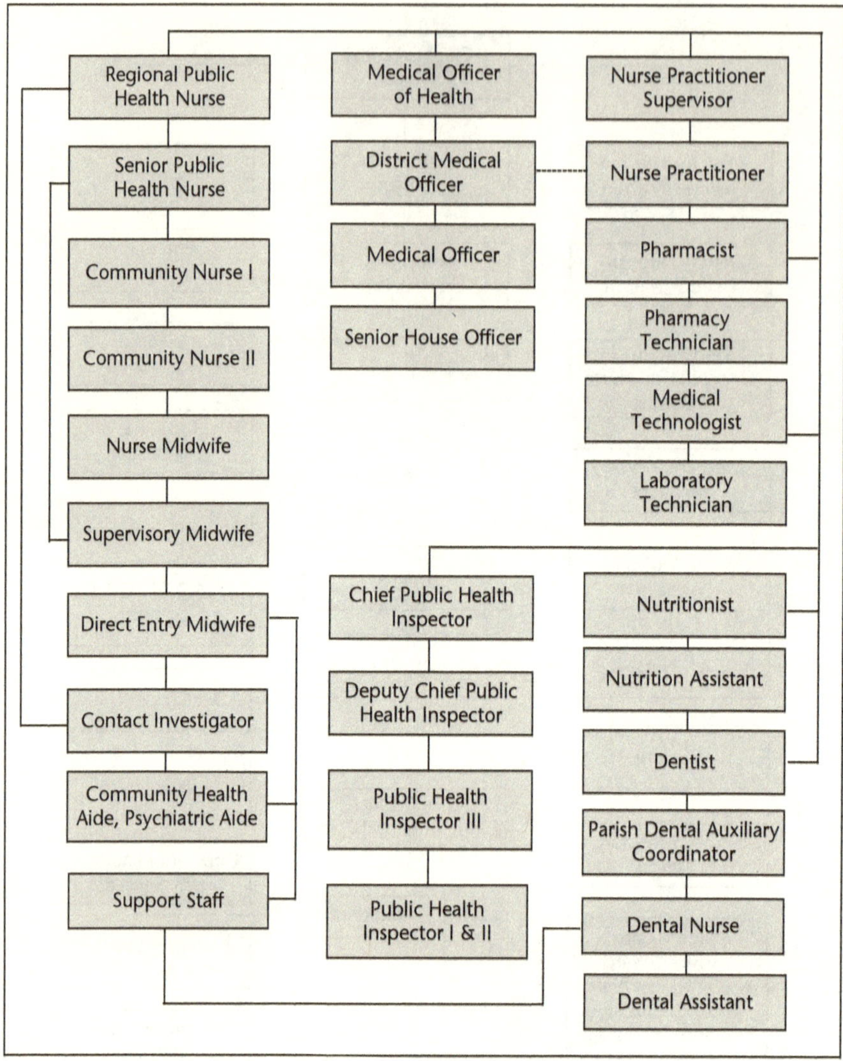

Figure 6. Typical structure of a Primary Health Care System

NURSING CATEGORIES

Given this research is mainly focusing on the work of the professional nurse, a brief description of the nurses' main categories is provided. Categories include the staff nurse or Level I nurse, the specialist nurse or Level II nurse, the nurse manager or Level III nurse, the PHNs, and the NPs. Figure 7

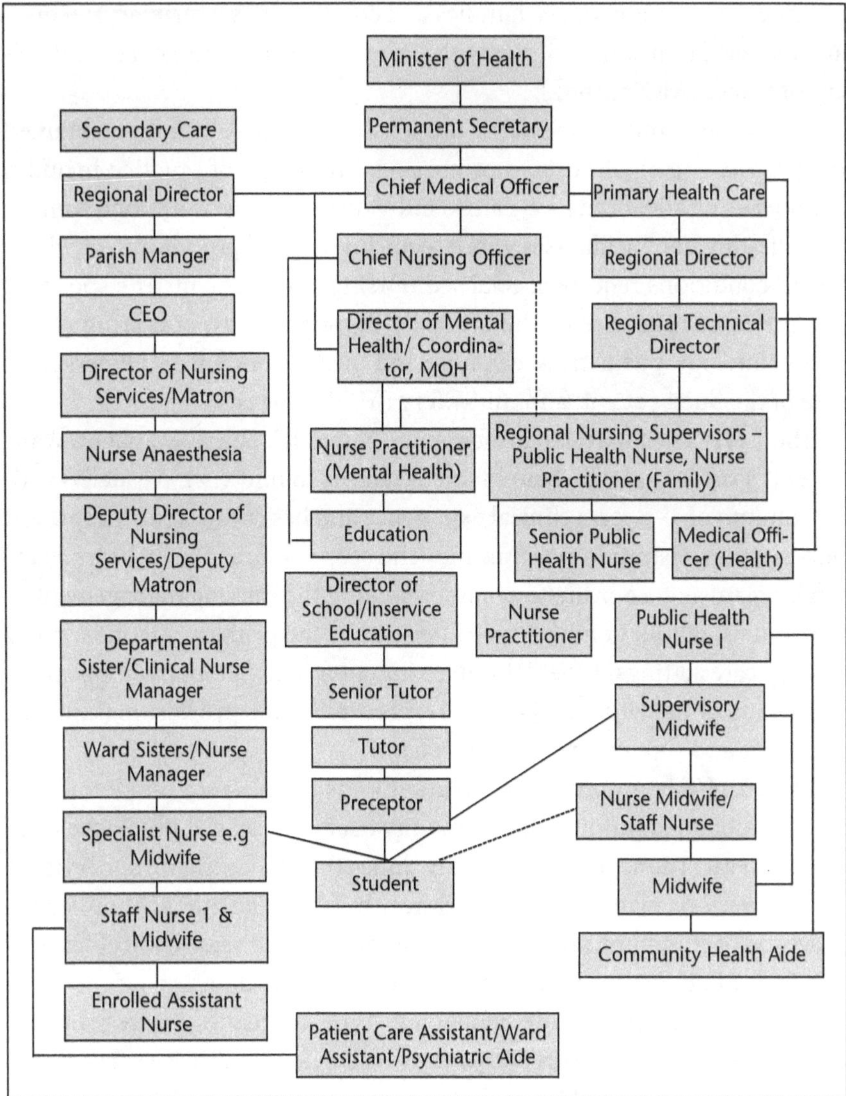

Figure 7. Nursing structure in the Public Health System

illustrates the nursing structure from MOH to hospitals and health centres. A Level I/Nurse I/Professional Nurse I is the entry-level professional nurse or staff nurse. As a new graduate, a staff nurse possesses the professional skills to practise within prescribed scope as a member of the health team. A staff nurse has direct and indirect responsibility for the nursing care and management of individuals, families and communities in primary, secondary and tertiary health facilities with the exception of intranatal care/delivery of babies (MOH, 1992).

A Level II nurse or specialist nurse is a staff nurse who has obtained training in a specialised field of nursing. The scope of practice includes administering advanced level care to individuals, families, and communities with life-threatening illnesses, those requiring surgical procedures, or whose health conditions require specialised nursing management. The specialist categories include care of the critically ill, nephrology, operating room, ophthalmology, paediatrics, ear, nose and throat, accident and emergency, care of the burn patient, and midwifery (MOH, 1992).

The Level III/Nurse III/Professional Nurse III/Nurse Manager/Ward Sister is a staff nurse who has obtained training in midwifery (usually) with a minimum of 5–7 years clinical experience and has completed an approved nursing administration programme. The scope of practice includes planning, organising, coordinating and evaluating the nursing management of individuals, families and communities within the primary, secondary and tertiary care settings. Level III nurses function in key leadership positions in various units with supervisory responsibility for professional nurses, midwives and support staff (MOH, 1992).

The PHN/Community nurse I/Level IV is a registered nurse midwife who has obtained training in community health nursing at the Bachelor of Science level. The scope of practice includes the management, supervision and delivery of maternal and child health, family health, school health, provision of communicable and non-communicable disease control services within the PHC setting and some secondary care facilities.

Additional roles include managing Type II health centres, having oversight for Type I centres and active involvement in disease surveillance and investigations (MOH, 1992).

The NP/Level V is a registered nurse/midwife or certified mental health nurse with five years clinical experience who has obtained a Master of Science degree in Family Nurse Practitioner, mental health/psychiatric nurse practitioner or other specialty. The scope of practice includes provision of nursing medical and mental health/psychiatric care to individuals, families and communities as legally permissible. NPs practise in advanced roles and conduct physical/mental examinations of a medical nature, make medical diagnoses, order laboratory and other investigations, interpret find-ings of these investigations and prescribe medications according to standing orders. Prescribing rights are currently being negotiated for NPs. They work parallel to the doctors in PHC and are sometimes found in secondary, tertiary and extended care settings (MOH, 1992). A CNO has overarching responsibility for professional nursing and midwifery services in the country and advises the government on nursing and midwifery issues. The CNO's post is within the MOH and reports to the CMO.

The public health system is faced with a chronic shortage of all categories of nurses. Reports have revealed that in 2008 only 53.0% of the required 244 of public health nurses were in the public health system, with registered nurses at 74.0% of the required 2547. The number of midwives was also low at 54.0% of the required 528. This trend is likely to worsen with the annual attrition rate of 15.0% (Watson & Williams, 2008, MOH personnel, personal communication, November 16, 2012). This has serious implications for access and the delivery of quality services to consumers.

UTILISATION OF HEALTH SERVICES

The choice between public and private health facilities is often influenced by people's perceptions of the quality and efficiency of the services provided. Other factors known to influence the choice of health facility include distance from the facility, availability of transport, diversity of the service, how technologically advanced the service is, operating hours, cost of the service, access to health insurance, preference and the severity of the illness (MOH, 2009).

Despite the aforementioned factors, many people (especially the poor) mainly utilise the public health facilities. Public sector hospitals continue to be the leading providers of hospital-based care, whereas the private sector is the leading provider of pharmaceuticals, laboratory services, radiographic services and ambulatory services (MOH, 2008b). Some utilisation patterns in the public health system are highlighted below, using pre-reform data from the MOH 2007 Annual Report. Although there were slight variations in utilisation over the period 2003-2007, the patterns were fairly consistent, as shown in Tables 7 & 8.

Table 7: Total health centre and curative visits: 2003–2007

Year	Health Centre Visits			Curative Visits		
	Total	**Male**	**Female**	**Total**	**Male**	**Female**
2003	1,586,630	480,635	1,105,995	695,125	232,605	462,520
2004	1,535,530	463,592	1,071,938	669,398	220,390	449,008
2005	1,514,415	459,889	1,054,526	654,658	217,683	436,975
2006	1,525,680	464,017	1,061,663	677,435	226,942	450,493
2007	1,490,844	455,171	1,035,673	674,162	226,477	447,685

Source. Adapted: *Ministry of Health, Jamaica (2009). Annual Report 2007.* Kingston, Jamaica: Author

Table 8: Attendance and source of referral to public Casualty Departments: 2003–2007

Year	Total Visits	Total Receiving care	Total Referral		Referral Source				
				Self	**Private Doctor**	**Health Centre**	**Police**	**Other Hospital**	**Other**
2003	746,844	727,977	693,048	88.3%	1.7%	2.0%	2.0%	1.1%	5.0%
2004	775,727	758,835	714,447	88.7%	1.8%	1.8%	1.6%	1.0%	5.0%
2005	694,354	682,009	638,830	87.4%	1.8%	1.8%	1.8%	1.2%	6.0%
2006	715,707	702,783	661,835	88.0%	1.8%	1.8%	1.8%	1.1%	5.5%
2007	785,284	765923	750,930	85.6%	1.7%	1.8%	1.9%	1.2%	7.9%

Source. Adapted: Ministry of Health, Jamaica (2009). *Annual Report 2007.* Kingston, Jamaica: Author.

The report showed that utilisation of health centres had some fluctuation over time; nevertheless, curative services increased marginally in 2006 over 2004 and 2005. There was a 3.9% decline in health centre visits and 2.6% reduction in curative visits in 2006 in comparison to 2003. Additionally, when the data were disaggregated by gender, females were the most frequent users of the facilities. Generally, females accounted for 69.5% of the total number of health centre visits in comparison to 30.5% for males. This observation could be attributed to the fact that maternal and child health visits were subsumed under health centre visits and women were the usual attendees at these clinics (MOH, 2009).

During the same period of time there was a noticeable increase in the total number of visits to the public hospital casualty departments. The report also revealed that self-referral (88.0% in 2006) was the main source of referral to public hospitals' casualty departments (Table 8). While data for the sources of referral to PHC facilities were unavailable, it is likely that self-referral was also the main mode of referral (MOH, 2009).

HEALTH INDICATORS

Health indicators are often used to determine the health status of a nation. Frequently monitored indicators are birth and death rates (Table 9). While attempts have been made to capture the indicators, the data presented may not be accurate. This is because some individuals do not register births or deaths, or reports may not be completed in a timely manner (MOH, 2008b).

In addition to monitoring health indicators, examining the leading causes of death in a country is fundamental to health policy planning and implementation. In 2008 the three leading causes of death in Jamaica were external causes (such as sudden and violent causes reported by police), cerebrovascular diseases and diabetes mellitus (STATIN, 2010). When causes of death were disaggregated according to sex, the leading causes of death among males 2006–2008 were external causes. In contrast, the leading causes of death among females for the same period were cerebrovascular diseases (Table 10) (STATIN).

Table 9: Health indicators 2003–2007

Health Indicators	Years				
	2003	2004	2005	2006	2007
Life Expectancy at Birth (Years)	74.13	74.13	74.13	74.13	74.13
Contraceptive Prevalence (%)	68.80	69.10	69.01	69.01	69.01
Total Fertility Rate (per woman)	2.5	2.5	2.5	2.5	2.5
Crude Birth Rate (per 1,000 mean population)	19.30	17.60	17.25	17.04	17.00
Crude Death Rate (per 1,000 mean population)	6.00	6.30	6.10	5.70	6.40
Infant Mortality Rate (per 1,000 live birth)	19.90	19.90	19.90	19.90	21.30
Child <5 years mortality rate (per 1,000 live births)	n/a	n/a	31.30	32.00	25.40
Maternal Mortality Ratio (per 100,000 live births) (hospital-based)	106.20	106.20	94.80	94.80	94.80

Source. Adapted: Ministry of Health, Jamaica (2009). *Annual Report 2007.* Kingston, Jamaica: Author

Table 10: *Ten leading causes of death among males and females in Jamaica: 2006-2008*

Cause of death – males	2008	2007	2006
External Causes*	1, 984	2, 065	1,464
Cerebrovascular Diseases	873	878	772
Diabetes Mellitus	630	671	633
Malignant Neoplasm of Prostate	544	589	522
Ischaemic Heart Diseases	476	543	511
Hypertensive Diseases	449	436	393
Chronic Lower Respiratory Diseases	337	336	310
Other Heart Diseases	332	352	335
Malignant Neoplasm of the Larynx, Trachea, Bronchus	321	284	305
Human Immunodeficiency Virus (HIV) Disease	247	233	235
Total	**6,193**	**6,387**	**5,480**

Cause of death – females	2008	2007	2006
Cerebrovascular Diseases	1,135	1,131	969
Diabetes Mellitus	1,079	1,017	1,063
Hypertensive Diseases	588	631	514
Ischaemic Heart Diseases	500	549	521
External Causes*	349	342	216
Other Heart Diseases	347	363	309
Other Malignant Neoplasm	294	329	263
Malignant Neoplasm of the Breast	257	252	228
Human Immunodeficiency Virus (HIV) Disease	180	164	156
Malignant Neoplasm of the Cervix Uteri	142	164	133
Septicaemia	142	72	62
Total	**5,013**	**5,014**	**4,434**

*External causes include sudden and violent cases reported by the police but not yet registered by the Registrar General's Department

Source. Adapted: STATIN. (2010). *Demographic Statistics 2009.* Kingston, Jamaica: Author

CHAPTER 5

Patient's Journey in Accessing Health Care Services

Understanding the manner in which users gain entry into a health facility is important, and a brief description is given here of what embodies the patient's journey in accessing the health services. The journey to accessing health services varies among institutions, as well as according to the nature of a user's health condition. Figure 8 describes the typical pathway to accessing a General Practitioner (GP), hospital or health centre. On entering the facility of choice, the process usually follows some organised manner. For example, there would be an initial registration, which entails a cost, then triaging to determine the level of treatment required. Once the treatment modality is determined the patient is either treated and discharged, referred, or admitted for further management.

While the typical pathway is widely-known and accepted, it is important to mention the alternative pathways frequently adopted to obtain non-conventional modes of treatment. It is not uncommon for individuals across the socio-economic spectrum to concomitantly utilise conventional and non-conventional modes of treatment for their health conditions. Self-medication with medicinal herbs is embedded in the Jamaican culture and was found to be prevalent among retirees and individuals 65 years and over (Picking, Younger, Mitchell, & Delgoda, 2011). In 2009, 49.0% of persons reported using home remedies for their illness instead of seeking care (PIOJ & STATIN, 2010).

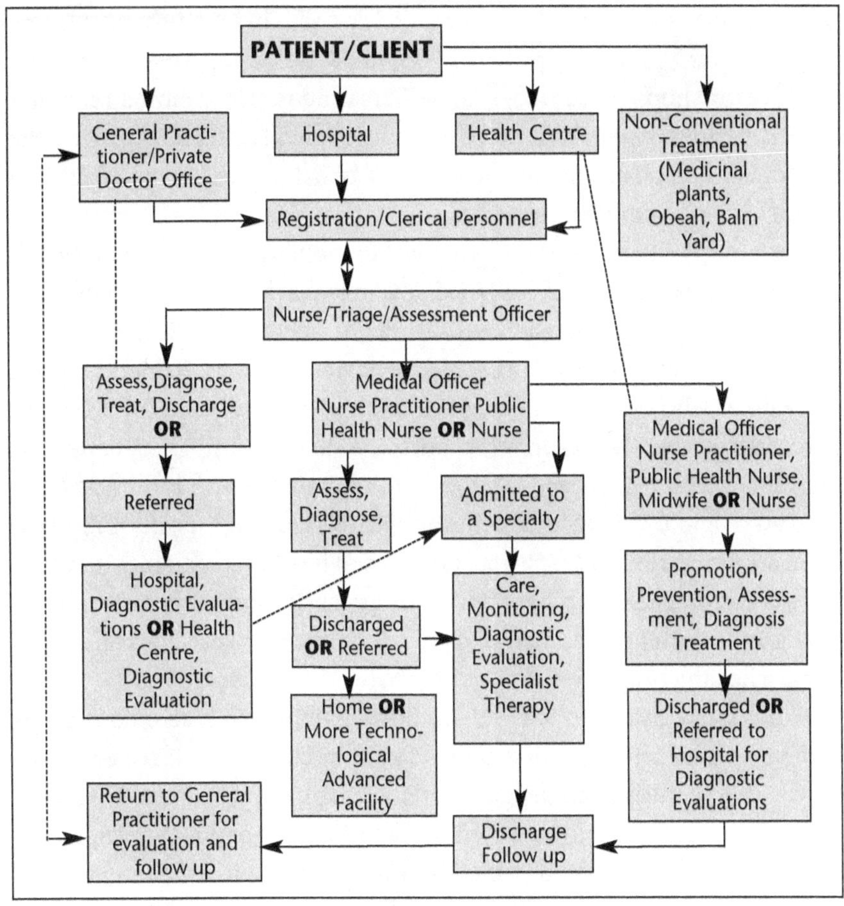

Figure 8. Patient's journey to accessing health care

FOLK CULTURE AND HEALTH-SEEKING BEHAVIOUR

Culturally, elements of African ancestry are threaded throughout the Jamaican experience. This is evident in the country's language, belief system and religion. There is also a strong link between health-seeking behaviours and African traditions, of which folk medicine remains a popular choice. Despite the advancement in scientific medicine some Jamaicans continue to adopt various forms of traditional healing practices or folk medicine for their ailments (Seaga, 2005; Weaver, 2003). This practice is not confined to any particular socioeconomic group and is present in both urban and rural communities. Common practices included obtaining treatment from the "doctor shop" (pharmacy) for self-treatment, use of home remedies especially those made from herbs and medicinal plants, and engaging the services of herbalist, spiritual healers and 'obeah man/woman', albeit in a clandestine manner (Seaga; Weaver).

It is also true to say that the spiritual component of sickness and health is integral to the practice of Folk medicine in Jamaica and its use is not influenced by religious persuasion. Additionally, belief in African spirits has strongly influenced health-seeking behaviour and is evident among individuals who seek treatment at the 'balm yard' for diseases or problems perceived to be the result of a curse. A 'balm yard' is operated by revival/spiritual healers and is a form of Pukumina, which is derived from African religion. Connecting with the spirit world and the gift of discernment are key attributes of spiritual healers and healing ceremonies may take several forms, including baptism, bathing, sprinkling of rum, 'read-up', purification with fire, and herbal drinks and other concoctions considered to have healing properties.

Healers may also give their patients prescriptions. While ceremonies may be held in a 'balm-yard', they are also held in churches, offices or public spaces. The venue is often dependent on the nature of the illness. Therefore, it may be on holy (usually in a church) or ordinary ground (Weaver, 2003). Ceremonies are often accompanied by invocation of spirits through singing and beating of drums. In addition, paraphernalia such as consecrated water, bottles of wine and white rum, candles, frankincense and myrrh, herbs and other concoctions are used to achieve spiritual healing. Faith plays a significant role in obtaining the desired effects from spiritual therapy (Seaga, 2005).

CONCLUSION

Undoubtedly, the Jamaican public health system has demonstrated resilience over time, responding to changes in the country's social, economic, and political situations. Several policy directives consistent with national priorities have been promulgated. As a result, the Jamaican health service has seen an expansion of the public health system in the post-independence period; contraction under the IMF structural adjustment programme, which resulted in shortage of resources, staff-cuts, closure and downsizing of health facilities and attrition of health personnel such as nurses; changes in modes of funding of the public health system; re-introduction of user fees; training of new cadres of health practitioners; decentralisation and the establishment of RHAs; and the abolition of user fees in 2007 and 2008. These reforms have had significant impacts on the health system.

Despite the promulgation of Acts, the appointment of commissions and implementation of various reform processes to improve efficiency and effectiveness in the public health system, poor access to health services remains a problem for some people; the system is underfunded; and the cadre of health workers, especially nurses, remains deficient.

CHAPTER 6

The Abolition of User Fees in the Jamaican Public Health System during the 21st Century

Stakeholders' Perceptions

The impact of the abolition of user fees in the Jamaican public health system was evaluated in 2010 utilising a multi-layered, mixed methods approach. Data were obtained from three perspectives: policymakers, practitioners and users. The main objective of the policy change was to improve access to health services for all Jamaicans, with the expectation that people who had deferred care because of costs would now access the services. Evaluating the impact of the policy change one year after its implementation in 2009 may be viewed as too soon, since any change in the system might not yet have been appreciable. However, it is clear that changes to the public health system were apparent as soon as the policy was implemented and this study captured the early days of the policy, including the implementation process and issues that required attention.

OVERALL IMPRESSION OF THE POLICY CHANGE

Policymakers. The stakeholders involved in this study had varied impressions of the policy. Policymakers were very positive and keen on setting up systems parallel to other countries with similar policy changes to ensure sustainability of the policy. A possible explanation for such optimism could be that there had been no official evaluation of the policy, despite some practitioners publicly expressing concerns about the negative effects of the policy.

Practitioners. Practitioners were desirous of having the system revisited and possibly reversed. They were more interested in a targeted system rather than universal system. Opinions voiced by practitioners included the following: (a) the policy should have been implemented on a phased basis; (b) free health services should only be available to children and the elderly; (c) a basic package should be created whereby persons would pay for more sophisticated tests; (d) a zoning system should be introduced to limit users to a particular geographic area, in order to control roving users who were sometimes triple-dipping in terms of pharmaceuticals; (e) those who can afford to should pay out-of-pocket for services; and (f) those with health insurance should be required to use their insurance. The current arrangement did not allow holders to use their health insurance to access health care in the public system.

There was no shortage of criticism of the policy change from practitioners, who felt the policy had been poorly executed and required revisiting. Some described it as a failure, making references to the lack of funding and increased risk of compromising the services being offered to the users. The reason behind practitioners being so critical of the policy change may be due to them being at the operational level and strategically positioned to evaluate the extent to which the policy was working. Furthermore, their work had been acutely affected by the policy change.

Users. Amidst policymakers' optimism and main health practitioners' discontent, there was a high level of satisfaction among the users who were the greatest beneficiaries. The study found that the users surveyed were satisfied with the new system, despite voicing concerns about the challenges they encountered while trying to access health care services.

Monitoring. No specific system for monitoring the policy had been established. This resulted in reliance on existing systems, which may not have been an efficient mechanism to capture those changes associated with the new policy. This has implications for recognising the changes and addressing problems in a timely manner. Ineffective monitoring may also affect the success of the policy.

IMPACT OF THE ABOLITION OF USER FEES ON ACCESS TO HEALTH SERVICES

To fully understand the study's results in terms of access, the perception of policymakers, practitioners and the users on access and availability of resources since the policy change, was taken into consideration. While the findings regarding increased utilisation of the health facilities are unequivocal, it is pertinent to discuss the findings regarding the other dimensions to access, because increased utilisation is dependent on people's ability to gain entry into the health system.

How is access defined from the users' perspective? Based on the findings, users' interpretation of this concept might not be clear-cut, because there were reports that access to health services was easier since the policy change despite people having to wait in long queues at the pharmacy, in treatment rooms and for surgical procedures. For users, having to wait to be seen was less of an issue than receiving the medications and treatment. Reports by some users, practitioners and policymakers indicated that access to health services such as pharmaceuticals was particularly problematic. There were issues with buying drugs at private pharmacies, having to pay for the drugs that were not on the VEN list at government pharmacies, only being able to purchase a portion of the prescribed medications, foregoing prescribed drugs generally, and waiting until medication was available at the government pharmacy. Many users were not holders of health insurance and, while some had a National Health Fund card, access to medications and health care generally was still a challenge. Therefore, an increase in the number of people visiting the health facilities may not translate into improved access to health services.

It is apparent that the drug supply issues in Jamaica were two-fold. First, the supply of drugs was inadequate, and, second, expensive drugs were not on the VEN list. This has implications for the procurement of drugs and revision of the VEN list. Although a number of measures were taken by the Jamaican government including expanding the VEN drug list to provide access to more pharmaceuticals in government pharmacies, instituting a government card for easy access to drugs in private pharmacies, and procuring cheaper drugs in larger amounts from international agencies, more intervention is needed. For example, alleviating these problems in Jamaica might entail establishing a mechanism whereby only listed drugs are prescribed, expensive drugs are subsidised, or frequently prescribed expensive drugs are added to the list

Another important finding was that some users were roving between health facilities and would frequently hoard the drugs obtained at these facilities. The extent of this practice is not known. This finding was unexpected and suggests that users did not trust that the policy would be sustained and that more patient education is required regarding the purpose of the policy change, the use of pharmaceuticals, and the use of the health services in general. The lack of trust that the system would last may be attributed to the nation's historical background, one tainted with mistrust and oppression under Plantocracy. Double dipping in pharmaceutical supplies put additional financial strain on an already resource-constrained health system and was of concern to practitioners, who were unable to track patient records for continuity of care. To manage the problem, practitioners proposed a mechanism whereby standardised, centralised, and computerised systems would be established in all health facilities to track people's utilisation patterns.

In some countries such as Australia, tracking is managed by requiring people to present a unique identification card in order to access services. These cards, known as Low Income Earner or concession cards, enable holders to access subsidised services (Scott, 2001). The mechanism could also be used to prevent overuse of the system. A similar arrangement exists in Jamaica through registration with the NHF; however, it is available to all Jamaicans, not exclusively low-income earners, and has not been established or utilised as a tracking mechanism. Nevertheless, this arrangement entitles holders to subsidised drugs and could be adopted as a useful mechanism for tracking pharmaceutical uptake. The NHF could be reformed based on the Australian system as a mechanism to also improve access for the poor. This level of mobility among people has implications for policymakers to establish suitable mechanisms to address these problems for successful policy outcome.

New information was revealed in this study about access to helplines, telephones, out-of-hours services, and lack of resources in the facilities within the Jamaican context. Users were generally unsure about the availability of helpline or telephone facilities to assist them in obtaining assistance from a health professional. Although this lack of knowledge may be interpreted as a barrier to access, it is the researcher's belief that having access to helplines and telephones may not necessarily translate into better health-seeking behaviour. Other concerns raised by users included problems in accessing health services on weekends, public holidays and at night at some secondary care facilities, and the lack of resources (staff and equipment) generally. For these reasons, users adopted behaviours to cope with the issues, such as visiting private doctors for better and faster treatment. Access to helplines, telephones, and out-of-hours use of secondary care facilities are unreported. This finding, regarding some individuals reverting to the use of private facilities over public offerings, corroborates the JSLC 2009 report that investigated people's experiences since the abolition of user fees (PIOJ & STATIN, 2010). For some, the experience meant forgoing care when required, which was often linked to cost-related factors. Practitioners gave several accounts of users being sent away after initial assessment and asked to come back due to overcrowding and insufficient staff to address their health needs.

Nevertheless, users continued to visit these facilities for health care. The overcrowding did not deter users, who often changed their behaviour and queued up at health facilities very early in order to be seen. A possible explanation for the attitude toward such obstacles while accessing care is that users were not fully aware of what access constituted; therefore, visiting a health facility and being told to return for treatment on another day did not distort their perception of access. The finding about users being sent home because of overcrowding has not been previously described in other

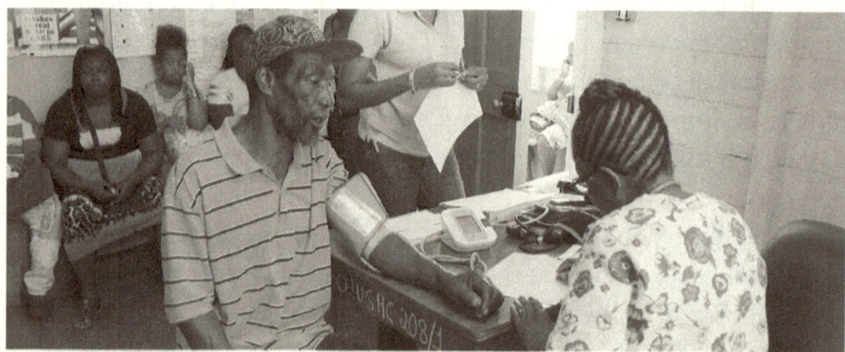

Overcrowding at health care facilities

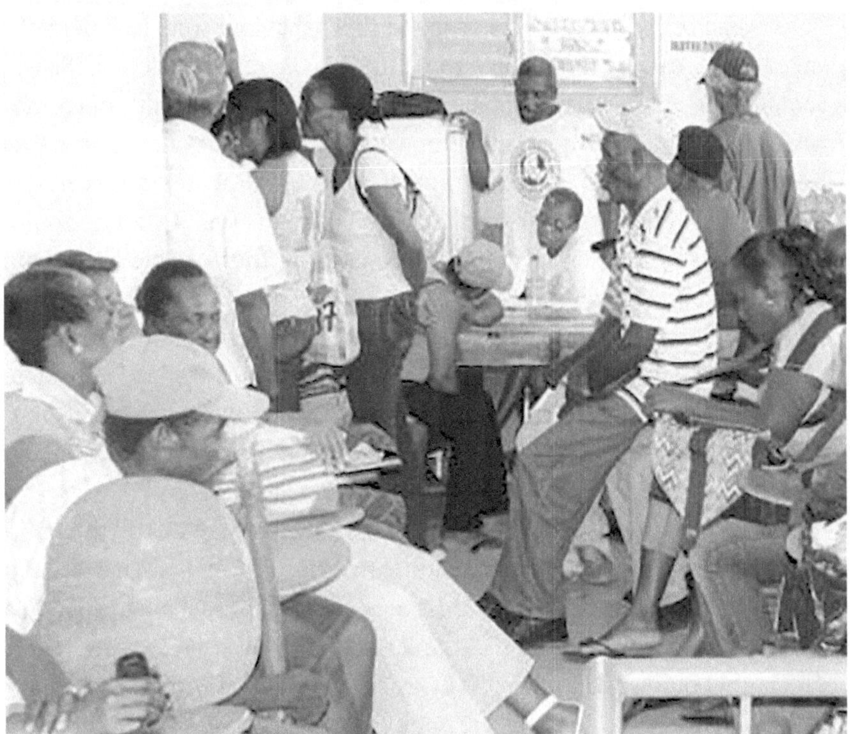

Overcrowding at health care facilities

research. This is an important finding because it is unclear how assessments or the decision regarding whom to send home was made, which may also indicate that people are experiencing other barriers to accessing health services. Returning home without being treated could result in worsened health conditions for the users.

The findings in this study revealed users were pleased that their expectations of the health system were being met. They were satisfied with the services provided and rated the quality of care received as good. Despite these favourable ratings and services now being free, the study confirmed some users continued to use alternative means of treatment such as home remedies, often in the form of bush tea; self-treatment; and the services of herbalists, spiritual healers, and traditional healers, whilst simultaneously obtaining treatment from health care facilities. There was no clear explanation for this finding; however, it is likely to be due to the cultural practices that embody Jamaican society.

Other factors possibly contributing to this behaviour were lack of confidence in the health system; belief that illness is the result of a curse (Seaga, 2005; Spence et al., 2010); or having had more positive health outcomes from alternative treatment in comparison to conventional treatments (Picking et al., 2011). While adopting self-care measures are positive health behaviours and consistent with international trends (WHO, 2002, 2008), the researcher, however, has concerns regarding the possible herb-drug interactions and efficacy of some treatments. Despite international (Ansah et al., 2009; Rutebemberwa et al., 2009) endorsement, the use of alternative medicines may produce undesirable health outcomes if inappropriately used. Therefore, this has implications for patient education; research into alternative treatments and their effects; and dialogue among stakeholders on the concomitant use of herbs and prescribed medications.

The need to travel far distances to access care may have contributed to the use of alternative or informal treatments, especially when transportation costs were a problem. Travelling across borders is often attributed to people's need to find facilities that offer all the services they need. Accordingly, policymakers should ensure all facilities are fully-equipped with the necessary resources to meet the needs of the population they serve. Travelling across borders also contributed to overcrowding in some facilities and disrupted continuity of care; therefore, measures should be implemented to enforce the use of services within particular borders. This recommendation endorses the suggestions by some participants to (1) institute zoning, and (2) introduce mobile services to make services more accessible to people.

While users were aware that user fees had been abolished, many were unable to identify all the services and drugs that were free. This suggests that some users were not knowledgeable about the package being offered to them and, therefore, may not have accessed some free services even if they had the need. This finding corroborates the report from the JSLC 2009, which found that some persons in the lower quintile were still not accessing care despite it being free. This could be attributed to people's lack of knowledge regarding the new service arrangements due to the precipitous nature of the policy change. Otherwise, it might be due to people's reluctance to learn about the details of the services available to them.

Dissemination of information about the policy in Jamaica was done via several channels, including print and electronic media, posters in health facilities, and health personnel. It is apparent that the dissemination of information process assumed some level of health literacy on the part of the users. It is also possible that those already engaged with the system had more exposure to the policy change than those who were not. The limited level of knowledge regarding free services is indicative of the need for further clarification of the policy for end-users. The findings have implications for a more targeted public education campaign regarding the terms and conditions of policies prior to implementation.

A large percentage of the users had been using the health facilities for protracted periods of time, which may explain the expressed levels of satisfaction with access to services, although there were concerns about lack of involvement in the planning of the services offered to them. Some users even travelled far distances to access the health facilities of their choice, which were not always the closest to their homes. Among the reasons given for their general choice of facilities were, good treatment, convenience, easy access both geographically and for appointments, and affordable services.

Additional costs for transportation and meals were incurred when individuals travelled far distances and waited long periods for care at health facilities. Equally, people who waited a long time for appointments, which could be over one year, were at risk of deteriorating health conditions that might require more extensive treatment, further adding pressure to the health system. These were cited as problems users encountered while accessing care. People were also frustrated and vented their feelings on the practitioners when they waited a long time for care. These findings suggest a need for alacrity in addressing the demand for resources that may result in reduced waiting times.

While no standardised instrument was used to capture the quality of services data, concerns raised by practitioners related to the limited time available to assess users due to the large number of persons; increase in dispensing errors since the policy change; inability to care for users holistically; and increase in users' complaints. The lens through which practitioners viewed these concerns might be explained in part by (1) the type of heath facility to which the practitioner was assigned, (2) the health outcomes of users since the policy change, (3) the staff complement at the facility, (4) whether the facility was rural or urban, (5) the level of teamwork in the facility, and (6) the availability of resources such as drugs.

The views, however, are invaluable since practitioners functioned at the operational level of the health facilities and had sufficient experience to judge the quality of services being offered. The inability to administer care according to expected standards not only jeopardised the lives of patients but also constituted additional stress for the practitioners and increased the likelihood of litigation. The threat of litigation was not explored in this study. Some practitioners were, however, concerned about their inability to deliver care in a manner consistent with their training, as well as the risk of losing their registration status. These concerns reflect the need for additional resources to ensure safe, effective and efficient service delivery. These findings are indicative of the need for policymakers to monitor quality indicators to ensure an efficient service delivery system.

This study found that there had been a reorienting of the Jamaican health system to accommodate the impact of the policy change. This included restructuring and strengthening the PHC system to reduce the pressure on secondary care services and promote preventive services. To accomplish this, health centres had been refurbished and new ones constructed, additional staff deployed to these areas, and people who utilised secondary services 'inappropriately' as suggested by practitioners, were frequently diverted to primary care facilities. Reorienting the public health system also meant training new categories of staff such as dialysis technicians, recruiting additional health practitioners locally and overseas, extending the opening hours, adjusting the shift system in some PHC facilities, and collaborating with private and semi-private organisations. These measures were adopted to ensure the efficiency of the public health system and success of the policy.

Policymakers felt that, in order to ensure access, other health-related policies could be implemented, for example, encouraging more self-care and introducing mobile-type services to alleviate problems associated with transportation when care was required. They were interested in improving services for particular population groups such as the elderly, adolescents and persons affected by HIV and AIDS. By the same token, others were concerned with policies that would foster utilisation of PHC facilities for non-emergency problems rather than A&E, with a caveat that the infrastructural arrangements in the PHC facilities would need to be improved.

Expanding the scope of practice for some health practitioners such as NPs, pharmacy technicians and patient care/ward assistants and clarifying the 40-hour work week were other means suggested by policymakers to make services more accessible to persons. While these proposals augur well for the policymakers, the impact of such interventions on health care delivery should be carefully assessed. These mechanisms, if addressed, would serve dual purposes. They could further improve users' access to health services, and avert any deleterious effects on staff. Health system modifications of this nature to improve access have not been mentioned in previous studies on the abolition of user fees.

Even though access to health services was a problem for some persons, self-referral was the main mode of entry to the health facilities by individuals requiring care. This suggests people were empowered to exhibit positive health-seeking behaviour. The mix of services also meant that people initiated and accessed care at various health facilities. This study found a slight increase in self-referral for 2009 in comparison to 2006 (Table 11). This

Table 11. Modes of referral to Casualty in 2006 & 2009

				Modes of referral				
Region	Year	Total referral	2006–2009 Increase (%)	Self	Hospital	Health Centre	Private Doctor	Other (including police)
MOH	2006	661,835		88.0%	1.1%	1.8%	1.8%	7.3%
	2009	891,281	35.0	88.5%	1.1%	2.0%	1.2%	7.1%
NERHA	2006	138,157		78.5%	0.4%	0.8%	0.5%	19.8%
	2009	184,290	33.4	82.7%	0.3%	0.7%	0.3%	16.0%
SRHA	2006	178,526		92.3%	0.6%	1.5%	2.2%	3.5%
	2009	245,454	37.4	85.6%	1.7%	2.7%	1.3%	8.8%
WRHA	2006	149,773		93.0%	0.9%	1.7%	1.4%	3.0%
	2009	209,644	40.0	95.0%	0.7%	1.5%	0.9%	1.9%
SERHA	2006	195,379		86.9%	2.2%	3.0%	2.7%	5.2%
	2009	251,893	29.0	90.2%	1.5%	2.7%	2.1%	3.5%

Source: Ministry of Health (2007). *Annual Report 2006.* Kingston, Jamaica: Author.
Ministry of Health (2009). *Annual Report 2007.* Kingston, Jamaica: Author.
Ministry of Health. (2010). *Annual Report 2009.* (Unpublished, Preliminary report). Kingston, Jamaica: Author.

increase may be attributed to the lack of gatekeeping in accessing health services, acceptance of self-referral as the main mode of entry into the health system, freedom to access care based on preference, and greater awareness of health needs under the new service arrangement. Gatekeeping by practitioners in primary care can reduce demand on hospital services (Forrest, 2003).

SOCIOECONOMIC GROUP AND IMPACT OF ABOLITION OF USER FEES

While this study did not categorically identify the socioeconomic status of who was utilising the services, several conclusions can be drawn from the data. Very low monthly incomes were reported by the majority of the users who completed the patient survey. Policymakers and practitioners reported that they considered the poor were benefiting from the policy change and that persons who had not been able to afford the services prior to the abolition of user fees were now accessing these services. Additionally, reports of an emerging trend whereby discharged users remained on the wards as borders for longer than necessary because family members chose not to receive them or continue their care at home are also indicative of the low socioeconomic status of people using the services.

While these accounts offer a suitable explanation for the socioeconomic status of the persons utilising the system, caution must be exercised in interpreting them. This is because the observed increase could also be attributed to what some practitioners described as an increase in the number of users being referred from private institutions since the policy change, as well as inappropriate use of the health facilities by some users. Of note is that some doctors working in the public sector also worked in private health facilities and it appeared that, since the policy change, they were now frequently referring their private patients to the public facilities. In addition to increasing the patient load, this suggests diversity in the social status of the users. People remaining in some Jamaican hospitals because families did not take them home coupled with reports of low income may be indicative of users' social status. Nevertheless, appropriate measures need to be established by policymakers to determine who is actually benefiting from the policy change, as this has implications for sustainability of the policy, future policy direction, and access.

IMPACT ON UTILISATION OF HEALTH SERVICES

Utilisation increased following the removal of user fees. Reports by policy-makers, practitioners, and users corroborated data from the MOH and RHAs annual reports, showing increases in the following areas: hospital admissions, outpatient visits, A&E department visits, pharmacy utilisation, and health centre visits, as well as the total number of surgeries performed one year after the abolition of user fees.

MOH data showed that, there was an increase in the total number of new cases in 2009 over 2006 (MOH, 2010). Analysis of this data however, indicates that those persons using the services were mostly repeat users, returning for treatment for the same or new illnesses. This was deduced from the number of years people had been using the system. This may not be a true reflection of increased access. This raises a very important issue concerning people who might be ill yet still not accessing the required care, as well as others who may have reverted to the use of private facilities and other modes of treatment, a finding which is supported by the JSLC 2009 (PIOJ & STATIN, 2010). Noteworthy is that utilisation in Jamaica declined six to nine months after the implementation of the policy, which suggests that the significant initial increase may have been due to gaps in the system, people who were ill having delayed seeking care prior to the policy change, or people possibly being disenchanted with overcrowding in the facilities.

The findings, however, regarding the decline in utilisation after implementation of the policy occurred at varying time periods. Despite the reported decline, the study revealed sustained daily overcrowding at the health facilities. This has implications for health practitioners' workloads and levels of satisfaction, as well as for the supply of resources.

REGIONAL VARIATION IN UTILISATION OF SOME SERVICES

Regional variations were evident in the manner in which people utilised the services. Most diabetics accessed hospital in-patient care in the NERHA (the smallest region) whereas most of those accessing PHC facilities did so in the largest region, SERHA. People affected by hypertension accessed care in PHC settings in SERHA generally. It is not possible to explain the regional variation in Jamaica from this research, however, this phenomenon may be due to several factors including users' preference of facility, the manner in which facilities offer services, people in an acute state seeking care from hospitals rather than PHC, PHC users possibly having better health-seeking behaviours and being more aware of the services available to them; or supportive follow-up systems in the health institutions.

Data obtained from the MOH and RHAs' annual reports revealed there was an overall increase in the Maternal and Infant Mortality and Crude Death rates in 2009. Three regions (SRHA, WRHA, and SERHA) recorded a decreased Infant Mortality rate. The increase in the crude death rate, however, was across all four RHAs. Also found was an overall increase in Maternal Mortality rates generally, with marked increases in SRHA and SERHA. The changes in Maternal Mortality rates might not necessarily be associated with the policy change, as they might be influenced by demographic changes, as well as the recording mechanisms used by the MOH and RHAs. Nevertheless, the high maternal mortality rate recorded in SRHA is of concern and requires further examination to establish the contributing factors. As alluded to earlier, in the absence of analyses to take into account any confounding variables, there are no clear explanations for these unanticipated findings. These results should, therefore, be interpreted judiciously as they have not been previously observed in other studies.

IMPACT ON THE WORK OF MAIN HEALTH PRACTITIONERS AND THE PROFESSIONAL NURSE

Main health practitioners' workload increased following the policy change. Practitioners embraced the policy change, although there was feeling of discontent about a number of issues such as their non-involvement in the policy process. This finding was endorsed by policymakers, who reported that the health workforce had embraced the policy and offered excellent service in some facilities even though they were pressured. Practitioners' concerns included feeling stressed and overburdened by the increased workload since the policy change. Such experiences, however, did not negatively affect their resolve to make the policy work. Practitioners' increase in workload may be the consequence of a number of factors: (a) additional workload not only from people genuinely in need of health care but also the inappropriate and haphazard manner in which other persons used the facilities, (b) having to

work and manage facilities with inadequate staff, and (c) having to impro-
vise in the face of limited resources in order to offer quality service. To
address this type of user behaviour, policymakers need to reinforce existing
measures and establish new ones in order to sensitise people about the
appropriate use of the different types of health services. Mechanisms to
ensure adherence to the measures should also be introduced.

As well as increased patient load, practitioners reported seeing existing
health conditions in larger numbers. For example, they were seeing more
users with chronic diseases such as hypertension, diabetes and lung disorders, rather than new conditions. This finding suggested that the case mix
had remained the same for most facilities and existing users were utilising
the services more often. These findings suggest that the profile of the users
of the Jamaican health system since the policy change needs more targeted
investigation.

RESOURCES AND THE WORK OF MAIN HEALTH PRACTITIONERS

Compounding the increase workload of practitioners were a number of
other factors including under-equipped facilities, lack of computerised systems in some pharmacies, and poorly-functioning equipment. While the
experience with equipment may be related to untimely maintenance, it may
also be due to the additional strain from the increased demand and the low
priority given to repair equipment by policymakers due to a shift in focus
to other matters. The claim regarding resources resonated with both policymakers and practitioners. Supplies such as family planning methods and
reagents for diagnostic tests were inadequate. Practitioners were often frustrated because of their inability to provide the services required; in some
circumstances users were asked to purchase their own materials in order to
access procedures such as hernia repair. This finding revealed that only
some users could afford to purchase materials and, as such, inequities continued in the system. Equally, poor access to family planning methods pre-
disposes a childbearing family to unplanned pregnancies, STIs and
economic hardship. Patients having to pay out-of-pocket for supplies, indicates that the policy, which was meant to improve access, was now creating
barriers and inequity.

Of significance is that this study found practitioners changed the manner in which they offered care in order to contribute to improving access to health care services. Changes included extending health facilities' working days and working hours; adjusting some institutions' policies, especially those related to when and where staff would work; financially assisting users to obtain diagnostic procedures; patient education and additional pressure to complete duty schedules/rosters with the limited staff; collaboration with other units such as pharmacies; and new measures by which to monitor discharged users. Some amount of lobbying was also underway to obtain well-needed equipment such as CT scanners and MRI machines. It is apparent that practitioners were committed to making the policy work.

There was, however, a lack of appropriate casual space for some staff and as such, staff often had to take their lunch breaks at their workstations in the presence of waiting users. These users were sometimes 'abusive' and 'insensitive' to the needs of the practitioners. One explanation for these attitudes is that sometimes users would arrive at the facilities at very early hours of the morning and by lunchtime had already waited for long periods of time prior to receiving care. Of note is that some institutions made efforts to provide rest areas for staff. This finding suggests that practitioners' working conditions require more in-depth investigation. Measures by policymakers to maintain practitioners' health in order to enhance effective performance on the job are important. Satisfaction is paramount to retaining practitioners in the system and, as such, should receive the required attention.

In regards to staffing, policymakers alluded to an increase in staff for some health facilities; however, practitioners were of a different view, since the perennial shortage of staff prior to the policy change had still not been sufficiently addressed. As a result, practitioners were now working longer hours sometimes without lunch or bathroom break periods. The increased working hours and lack of breaks resulted in staff experiencing health conditions such as digestive disorders and UTIs. While it may not have been effective, minimal work had initially been done to improve staffing in Jamaica. Efforts were made post implementation to recruit and train some categories of staff, for example, pharmacists and dialysis technicians, in order to boost the complement in the facilities (MOH, 2008b). These measures were intended to alleviate the pressure on the staff in the facilities, make the services available to users and maintain the quality of services provided, as well as minimise waiting times.

Despite there being several possible explanations, the aforementioned issues could be attributed to the limited budgetary support injected into the system prior to the policy change and the hurried nature in which the policy was implemented. Regional policymakers and practitioners considered the public health system to be underfunded and felt this should have received serious attention prior to the implementation of the policy. The budgetary shortfall meant lack of basic supplies such as syringes and needles. National policymakers, on the other hand, reported that there had been additional budgetary support to offset the policy implementation. Evidently, this allocation was insufficient and policymakers need to mobilise more funds to address the demands resulting from the policy change.

The policy had not allowed sufficient time for the key stakeholders to be engaged fully in the process, a concern that resonated with most practitioners. They reiterated the point that the policy change would have been more effectively managed if they were involved throughout all the stages of the policy process. An important lesson here is that all stakeholders must be integrally engaged in all phases of the policy process if it is to achieve widespread credibility and sustainability. Although practitioners in Jamaica embraced the policy generally, it is important to note that they were trying to make the policy work under stressful and difficult circumstances. Practitioners were often disenchanted with the increased workloads, overcrowding, limited resources, poor working conditions, and reduced time for patient assessment. Reduced assessment time resulted in practitioners accommodating more patients. These opinions suggest that it is important for policymakers to address these issues in order to improve satisfaction among practitioners.

CONCLUSION

In brief, there were varied views among policymakers, practitioners and users about the impact of the policy change. Utilisation of services increased immediately following the policy change; however, there was an initial decline six to nine months after with a sustained increase over the pre-policy period. Access was improved for all, which can be viewed positively, nonetheless, the policy also had some downsides, which may be additional barriers encountered by users in an attempt to access health care services.

The main health practitioners interviewed for this study embraced the user fees policy, despite concerns about several issues such as lack of involvement in the policy process prior to implementation. Although the main health practitioners perceived that people were benefiting from the change, they also had concerns, which included the following: the health system's capacity to sustain the policy, increased workloads and overcrowding, poor working conditions, inadequate resources such as drugs and equipment, inadequate workspaces, misuse of the system and low morale.

References

Alleyne, D. (2010). The impact of user fees on health costs and health burdens in Jamaica: The cases of diabetes and hypertension. Social and Economic Studies, 59(1), 91-121,315-316,326. Retrieved from http://search.proquest.com/docview/749698043?accountid=14782

Ansah, E.K., Narh-Bana, S., Asiamah, S., Dzordzordzi, V., Biantey, K., Dickson, K., Whitty, C.J.M. (2009). Effect of removing direct payment for health care on utilisation and health outcomes in Ghanaian children: A randomised controlled trial. *PLoS Med, 6*(1), 48–58. Retrieved from http://search.proquest.com/docview/66861174

Bailey, W., Wynter, H.H., Lee, A., Oliver, P., & Jackson, J. (1994). The effect of user fees on the utilisation of family planning services. A clinical study [Abstract]. *West Indian Medical Journal, 43*(2), 43-5. http://www.ncbi.nlm.nih.gov/pubmed/7941495

Barrett, R.D., & Lalta, S. (2004). *Health financing innovations in the Caribbean*: EHPO and the National Health Fund. (Technical Papers Series). Washington, D.C:Inter-American Development Bank, Sustainable Development Department. Retrieved from http://www.eldis.org/vfile/upload/1/document/0708/DOC19862

Barnett, J., Lalta, S., & Bailey, W. (2010). Towards alternative financing proposals for health care for the elderly with chronic conditions – Jamaica. *Social and Economic Studies, 59*(1), 153-180,318-319,326-327. Retrieved from http://search.proquest.com/docview/749698273

Black, C. (2011). *History of Jamaica*. United Kingdom: Longman Group Publishing.

Bourne, P.A. (2009). Health insurance coverage in Jamaica: Multivariate analyses using two cross-sectional survey data for 2002 and 2007. *International Journal of Collaborative Research on Internal Medicine & Public Health, 1*(8), 195–213.

Campbell, C. (2002). Early emancipation Jamaica: The historiography of plantation culture, 1834–1865. In K. E. A. Monteith & G. Richards (Eds.), *Jamaica in Slavery and freedom:*

Heritage, history and culture (pp. 52–69). Kingston, Jamaica: The University of the West Indies Press.

Culture, Health, Arts, Sports and Education (CHASE) Foundation, Jamaica. (2008). Retrieved from http://www.chase.org.jm/

Cover, W.A. (1995). *Handbook of Jamaica 1955* (65th ed.). Ministry of Communications and Works. Kingston, Jamaica: Government Printing Office.

Figueroa, J.P. (2001). Health trends in Jamaica: Significant progress and a vision for the 21st century. *West Indian Medical Journal, 50* (Supplement 4), 15–22.

Flores, G., Abreu, M., Olivar, M.A., & Kastner, B. (1998). Access barriers to health care for Latino children. Archives of Pediatrics and Adolescent Medicine, 152, 1119–1125. Retrieved from https://mywebspace.wisc.edu/anoguera/web/med/Reading.for.class_11-02.pdf

Forrest, C. B. (2003). Primary care gatekeeping and referrals: Effective filter or failed experiment? *British Medical Journal, 326*(7391), 692–695. doi: 10.1136/bmj.326.7391.692

Gertler, P., & Sturm, R. (1997). Private health insurance and public expenditures in Jamaica. *Journal of Econometrics, 77*(1), 237–257. doi: 10.1016/s0304-4076(96)01814-3

Gordon-Strachan, G., Bailey, W., Henry-Lee, A., Barnett, J., Lalta, S., & Alleyne, D. (2010). The impact of user fees for preventive health care - Jamaica. *Social and Economic Studies, 59*(1& 2), 123–152. Retrieved from ://go.galegroup.com.helicon.vuw.ac.nz/ps/retrieve .do?retrieveFormat=PDF

Hay Ho Sang, E.P. (1985). *The development of nursing education in Jamaica, West Indies: 1900–1975.* Retrieved from ProQuest Dissertations & Theses. (Ann Arbor 48106).

Health Sector Task Force. (2007). *A healthy Jamaica in a healthy world.* Kingston, Jamaica: Ministry of Health & Environment.

Health Sector Task Force. (2009). *Vision 2030 Jamaica national development plan*: (Draft Health sector plan). Kingston, Jamaica: Ministry of Health & Environment.

Higman, B.W. (2005). *Plantation Jamaica 1750–1850: Capital and control in a colonial economy.* Kingston, Jamaica: The University of the West Indies Press.

Hussey, P., Anderson, G., Berthelot, J.M., Feek, C., Kelley, E., Osborn, R., Epstein, A. (2007). Trends in socioeconomic disparities in health care quality in four countries. *International Journal for Quality in Health Care, 20*(1), 53–61. doi: 10.1093/intqhc/mzmo55

Jamaica Information Service. (2008, March 11). Special attention being paid to primary health care system. Retrieved from http://www.jis.gov.jm/news/archive/14479

Kiwanuka, S.N., Ekirapa, E.K., Peterson, S., Okui, O., Hafizur Rahman, M., Peters, D., Pariyo, G.W. (2008). Access to and utilisation of health services for the poor in Uganda: A systematic review of available evidence. *Royal Society of Tropical Medicine and Hygiene, 102*, 1067–1074. doi:10.1016/j.trstmh.2008.04.023

Lewis, M.A. (1993). User fees in public hospitals: Comparison of three country case studies. *Economic Development and Cultural Change, 41*(3), 513-532. http://www.jstor.org/stable/1154314

McCaw-Binns, A. (2008). Can research accelerate progress toward Millennium Development Goal 5 (Maternal Health) in Jamaica? *West Indian Medical Journal; 57*(6): 549. Retrieved from http://dspace.mona.uwi.edu/handle/123456789/265

McCaw-Binns, A. M., Moody, C. O., & Standard, K. L. (1998). Forty years: An introduction to the development of a Caribbean public health. *West Indian Medical Journal, 47* (Supplement 4), 8–12.

McCaw-Binns, A., & Moody, C.O. (2001). The development of primary health care in Jamaica. *West Indian Medical Journal, 50* (Supplement 4), 6–10.

Ministry of Health. (1992). *Job descriptions (professional* nurses). Kingston, Jamaica: Author.

Ministry of Health. (2007). *Annual Report 2006.* Kingston, Jamaica: Author.

Ministry of Health. (2008a, March 28). *Statement on abolition of user fees in public health facilities.* [News release]. Kingston, Jamaica: Author

Ministry of Health. (2008b). *Annual report 2006.* Kingston, Jamaica: Author.

Ministry of Health. (2008c, March 28). *Question and answer sheet on abolition of user fees.* [News release]. Kingston, Jamaica: Author.

Ministry of Health. (2008d, April 9). *Successful first week for the abolition of fees with 58% increase in accident and emergency registration.* [News release]. Kingston, Jamaica: Author.

Ministry of Health. (2009). *Annual report 2007.* Kingston, Jamaica: Author

Ministry of Health. (2009a). *Patient utilisation one year after the abolition of user fees.* Retrieved from http://www.moh.gov.jm/general/latestnews/1-news?start=24

Ministry of Health. (2009b, February 24). *Jamaicans saved over 1 billion dollars under no user fees policy.* [News release]. Kingston, Jamaica: Author.

Ministry of Health. (2010). *Annual Report 2009.* (Unpublished, Preliminary Report). Kingston, Jamaica: Author.

Nabyonga, J., Desmet, M., Karamagi, H., Kadama, P., Omaswa, F., & Walker, O. (2005). Abolition of cost-sharing is pro-poor: Evidence from Uganda. *Health Policy and Planning, 20*(2), 100-108. doi: 10.1093/heapol/czio12

National Health Fund. (2008). *Aims and objectives.* Retrieved from http://www.nhf.org.jm/dynaweb.dti?dynasection=aboutus&dynapage=aims_objectives

National Health services Act 1997. Retrieved from http://www.moj.gov.jm/node/77

North East Regional Health Authority. (2009). Retrieved from http://www.nerha.gov.jm/aboutus.html

Pan American Health Organisation & World Health Organisation. (2007). *Jamaica. (Health in the Americas Volume II).* Retrieved from http://www.paho.org/hia/archivosvol2/

Picking, D., Younger, N., Mitchell, S., & Delgoda, R. (2011). The prevalence of herbal medicine home use and concomitant use with pharmaceutical medicines in Jamaica. *Journal of Ethnopharmacology, 137,* 305–311. Retrieved from http://www.tramil.net/files/Jamaican_survey.pdf

Planning Institute of Jamaica. (2011). *Economic and social survey Jamaica 2010*. Kingston, Jamaica: Author.

Planning Institute of Jamaica & Ministry of Foreign Affairs and Foreign Trade. (2009). *National report of Jamaica on Millennium Development Goals for the United Nations Economic and Social Council annual ministerial review*. Retrieved from PIOJ & STATIN. (2008). *Jamaica survey of living conditions 2007*. Kingston, Jamaica: Author.

Planning Institute of Jamaica & Statistical Institute of Jamaica. (2008). *Jamaica survey of living conditions 2007*. Kingston, Jamaica: Author.

Planning Institute of Jamaica & Statistical Institute of Jamaica. (2010). *Jamaica survey of living conditions 2009*. Kingston, Jamaica: Author. Public Health Act. (1985). Retrieved from http://www.moj.gov.jm/sites/default/files/laws/Public%20Health%20Act.pdf

Robertson, J. (2002). "Stories" and "Histories" in late seventeenth century Jamaica. In K.E.A.

Rutebemberwa, E., Pariyo, G., Peterson, S., Tomson, G., & Kallander, K. (2009). Utilisation of public or private health care providers by febrile children after user fee removal in Uganda. *Malaria Journal, 8*(1), 45. doi:10.1186/1475-2875-8-45

Safriet, B.J. (1992). Health care dollars and regulatory sense: The role of advanced practice nursing. *Yale Journal on Regulation, 9*, 417-488. http://www.lexisnexis.com.helicon.vuw.ac.nz/hottopics/lnacademic/?verb=sr&csi=7384

Sagicor Life Jamaica. (2012). Retrieved from http://www.sagicorjamaica.com/

Seaga, E. (2005). The folk roots of Jamaican cultural identity. *Caribbean Quarterly, 51*(2), 79–95. Retrieved from http://www.jstor.org/stable/40654507

Scott, C. (2001). Public and private roles in health care systems. Suffolk, UK: St Edmundsbury Press.

Shepard, D., Anthony, Y., McNaught, A., & Davis, K.L. (1998). *Evaluation of health sector program*. Prepared for USAID, Kingston, Jamaica. Retrieved from http://people.brandeis.edu/~shepard/j-eval3.PDF

South East Regional Health Authority. (2010). Retrieved from http://www.serha.gov.jm/ProfileRegion.aspx

Spence, D., Crath, R., Hibbert, A., Phillips-Jackson, K., Barillas, A., Castagnier, T., Webley, N. (2010). Supporting cancer patients in Jamaica – A needs assessment survey. *West Indian Medical Journal, 59*(1), 59–66

South Regional Health Authority. (2011). Retrieved from http://www.srha.gov.jm/RegionProfile.aspx

Statistical Institute of Jamaica. (2010). *Demographic statistics 2009*. Kingston, Jamaica: Author.

Swaby, G. (2005). *Profession of nursing*. Kingston, Jamaica: Stephenson's Litho Press Ltd.

Ward, E., & Grant, A. (2005). *Epidemiological profile of selected health conditions and services in Jamaica 1990–2002*. Kingston, Jamaica: Ministry of Health & Environment.

Warner Lewis, M. (2002). The character of African-Jamaican culture. In K.E.A. Monteith & G. Richards (Eds.), *Jamaica in slavery and freedom: Heritage, history and culture* (pp.

89–114). Kingston, Jamaica: The University of the West Indies Press.

Watson Williams, C. (2008). *Realising rights through social guarantees: The case of Jamaica.* Final Report submitted to the World Bank. Retrieved from http://siteresources.world-bank.org/EXTSOCIALDEV/Resources/3177394-1168615404141/3328201-1192042053459/Jamaica_fullReport.pdf?

Weaver, S.R. (2003). *Health and illness in a rural community: A study of traditional health care practices in the parish of St Thomas, Jamaica* (Unpublished PhD thesis). University of the West Indies, Mona, Kingston, Jamaica. [Email communication].

World Bank. (2011). World development indicators, Jamaica. International Bank for Reconstruction and Development/ The World Bank, Washington D.C. Retrieved from http://www.worldbank.org

Word Health Organisation. (2002). Traditional medicine strategy 2002–2005. Retrieved from http://whqlibdoc.who.int/hq/2002/WHO_EDM_TRM_2002.1.pdf

Word Health Organisation. (2008). Beijing declaration 2008. Retrieved from http://www.who.int/medicines/areas/traditional/TRM_BeijingDeclarationEN.pdf

Western Regional Health Authority. (2009). Retrieved from http://www.wrha.gov.jm/content/wrha_profile.html

West India Commission Report 1945. (2006). *House of Commons Parliamentary Papers online.* London, UK: ProQuest Information and Learning Company.

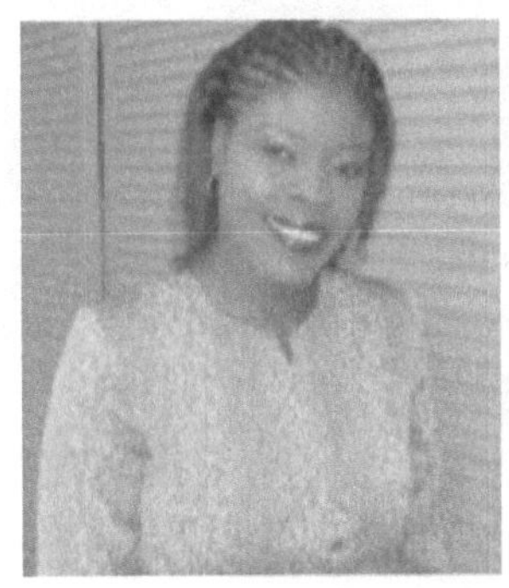

About the Author

From the mountainous farming community of Grant's Bailey in the Garden Parish of St Ann, as a child she was taken to James Hill in Clarendon where she spent most of her childhood and early teen years.

The desire to serve informed her decision to be trained as a Registered Nurse at the Kingston School of Nursing and subsequently to be posted at the May Pen Hospital. With training in midwifery added to her experience, she felt she could give more than just running wards and moved into nursing education.

She embarked on this aspect of her journey at the Kingston School of Nursing then the University Hospital of the West Indies School of Nursing after which she transitioned to the University of Technology (UTech), Jamaica in the Faculty of Health and Applied Sciences now the College of Health Sciences, Caribbean School of Nursing, UTech, Jamaica.

Dr Adella Campbell is a Justice of the Peace, an Associate Professor and Head of School at the Caribbean School of Nursing which has campuses in Papine and Braemar Avenue in Kingston and in Montego Bay. There are also two franchised sites, one at the Excelsior Community College in Jamaica and the other at the Community College in St Vincent and the Grenadines.

Becoming a Commonwealth Scholarship recipient took her to New Zealand and the Victoria University of Wellington from where she earned her PhD in Nursing.

She holds a Master of Science in Nursing Administration with distinction from the University of the West Indies (UWI); a BSc in Nursing Education with First Class Honours from UWI, and a Certificate in Nursing Education with Honours from UWI.

She is a Registered Nurse/Midwife by profession and also holds certification in Supervisory Management from the Jamaica Institute of Management and Industrial Relations and Negotiation Strategies from the Mona School of Business and Management.

She has a passion for research and is the only person to have undertaken indepth research into the much controversial decision by government to abolish user fees in the public health system.

She is presently involved in research and has presented at conferences locally, regionally and internationally.

Dr Campbell has earned several accolades from her place of work, for her voluntary contribution through Kiwanis and professional bodies. More recently, the Victoria University of Wellington, New Zealand, chose her to be the face of the university in its worldwide outreach.

PROFESSIONAL ORGANISATION:

- Dr Campbell is the executive chair for the CARICOM Network for Nursing and Midwifery Education
- Dr Campbell has served in different capacity in the Nurses Association of Jamaica including First Vice President, Key/Council member, Committee Chair and Committee member
- She has also served on Policy, Train Abroad and the Nursing and Midwifery Committees at the Nursing Council of Jamaica

EXTRA-CURRICULAR ACTIVITIES:

- Dr Campbell is involved in outreach projects through the Kiwanis Club of New Kingston and the Fellowship Tabernacle Church (Kingston).
- She served previously as Sunday School teacher, Youth Director and worked with Family Life and Women's Ministries at her church.

She enjoys:
- Coordinating activities such as social events and educational programmes
- Helping people, socialising and gardening

SOME FIRSTS:

- First and only Jamaican Nurse to be awarded the Commonwealth Scholarship
- Youngest Jamaican Nurse with a PhD in Nursing
- Contributor on nursing issues to the local paper *Jamaica Observer*

SPECIAL MEDIA FEATURES:

Dr Campbell was featured on the:

- Popular 'Profile' on Television Jamaica with Ian Boyne, 2013
- Television Jamaica morning programme *Smile Jamaica*, 2016
- Radio Jamaica Radio programme *Palav* with Gerry McDaniel, 2016
- She was also featured among the *Jamaica Observer* top 50 celebrated women in 2016 during *All Woman* 20th Anniversary celebration and as an outstanding alumni on the website of the Victoria University of Wellington, New Zealand, 2016
- She is the mother of one son.